TRAINING ATHLETES
FROM THE INSIDE OUT

---

*Yoga and Mindfulness Lesson Plans to
Reduce Stress and Enhance Performance*

Tawn Turnesa - Norton

Published by:

John Melvin Publishing, LLC

344 St. Joseph St.

Suite 538

New Orleans, LA 70130

www.johnmelvinpublishing.com

ISBN: 978-1-7351627-4-4 Paperback

Library of Congress Control Number: 2020923575

Printed in the United States of America

TABLE OF CONTENTS

DEDICATION

I never could have imagined that my initial curiosity about what "mindfulness" was would ultimately lead me to places I never knew existed. My perspective and attitude on life have completely changed since my immersion into mindfulness practices.

This book was inspired by my mindfulness journey that began in 2015 when I enrolled in mindful schools classes. It was followed by a year-long certification program which resulted in my certification as a mindful educator.

I want to thank all of my professors, mentors, and facilitators for inspiring me to continue this very important work in teaching others about the importance of living a mindful life. I would also like to thank Gia Weightman for providing all of the yoga stick figure images in this book.

FOREWORD

When I first met Tawn, she was presenting a workshop on mindfulness at a summer administrative retreat in my district. I knew from the moment I met her that she was a leader of mindfulness, champion of self-care, and someone I would learn and grow from in years to come.

In her role as Department Chair for Health & Physical Education, she has taught numerous classes promoting mindfulness and yoga to her students, peers, administrators, and families. She has also played an integral role in supporting the District Social Emotional Learning (SEL) initiative by creating lessons, sharing resources and demonstrating self-care practices to our school community. During COVID, Tawn co-lead weekly mindfulness calls with our teachers to help promote well-being and self-care during the turbulent times we were facing.

Training Athletes from the Inside Out is a resource that was written with the goal to provide coaches with resources to support their athletes with increasing their self-awareness, self-regulation, focus, positivity, and confidence in order to strengthen their core from the inside out.

Tawn has created an easy to follow, step by step guide that will help build the foundation for athletes of all ages with a focus on what they can control in order to become the best version of themselves. By training the body and the mind, athletes can perform at their peak performance and reach their highest potential.

The tips, tools, and techniques that are shared in this book will support athletes from the Inside-Out. It is a must read for all coaches!

Gail Duffy, Ed.D
Assistant Superintendent for Administration & Instruction
Public Schools of the Tarrytowns

INTRODUCTION

T his book will provide the reader with fifteen mini lessons to use once a week with his/her team either before or after a practice to increase self-awareness and encourage self-regulation of athletes' emotions. The lessons will consist of a fifteen to twenty-minute yoga session, a tip of the day, a focus/strategy of the day that will help reduce stress, and a five to ten-minute mindfulness exercise. I have also included sport-specific visualization scripts that can be used before games to help athletes increase their focus, positivity, and confidence going into a game.

Yoga will help athletes learn to move with their breath to create a mind-body connection, enhance their flexibility and strength, and achieve ultimate health and relaxation.

Mindfulness will help athletes become more self-aware, have improved attention & focus, and have better emotional regulation in their everyday life. It is all about learning how the mind works and how to retrain it to think more positively. As we have all heard, "Sports are 90% mental and 10% physical" (Meggyesy, 2016). That is why it is imperative that we not only train our bodies, but we train our minds as well.

When athletes can use both yoga and mindfulness together, they will find they have an increased ability to identify, express, and regulate their emotions in a healthy way. This internal awareness will help them create a more productive life and achieve greater focus while performing their sport.

LESSON ONE

Yoga

Sequence One:

Hands at heart – place palms together at chest level.

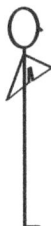

Mountain pose – circle the arms up, stand tall with the arms overhead parallel to the ears, shoulders relaxed and away from the ears, and feet hip distance apart.

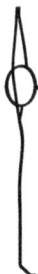

Forward hang - bend at the waist, reaching your arms and hands towards the floor. Hang forward with a relaxed head.

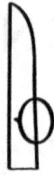

Shake head yes and no to release neck muscles.

Half lift – inhale, as you slide your hands along your shins with a straight back, upper torso coming up parallel to the ground; roll the shoulders back with the hands around the shins.

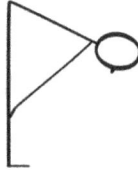

Forward hang – exhale, as you hang forward, reaching your hands towards the ground with a relaxed head.

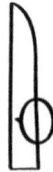

Downward dog – place your hands on the ground shoulder-width apart; step feet back hip-width apart; the body is in a V; press the hips up and press the chest towards the thighs; your head should be between your arms.

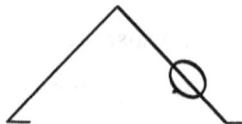

Walk the dog- pedal the heels, bending the right leg first and straightening the left, and then alternating to stretch the calves.

High plank – step the feet back with the toes on the ground, keep the body parallel to the floor, hands under shoulders, feet hip-width apart, core is tight, and shoulders are rolled back.

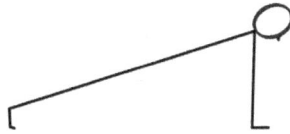

Lower yourself to the floor, leading with the chest and keeping your arms in, close to the body.

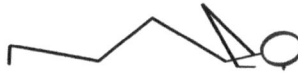

Upward dog - place hands at your sides at chest level, with the lower body on the floor; press into your hands and lift upper torso and hips off the ground; arms are straight, roll the shoulders back and look back for a slight backbend with the tops of the feet touching the ground.

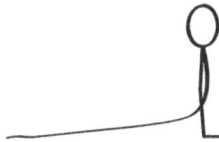

Downward dog – press back onto the balls of the feet with the feet hip-width apart; place your hands on the ground shoulder-width apart; the body is in a V; press the hips up and press the chest towards the thighs; your head should be between your arms.

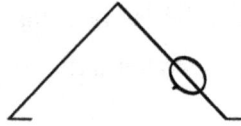

Forward hang - walk feet up, reaching your hands towards the floor for a forward hang.

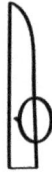

Mountain – stand tall with the arms overhead parallel to the ears, shoulders relaxed, and feet hip width apart.

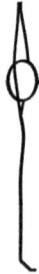

Repeat this sequence three more times starting with hands at heart

Sequence Two:

Mountain - stand tall with your feet hip-width apart, and your arms overhead parallel to your ears, shoulders relaxed and away from your ears.

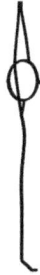

Forward fold - bend at the waist, reaching your arms and hands towards the ground. Hang forward with a relaxed head.

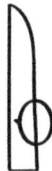

Left runners lunge – place your hands on the ground on either side of your left foot; step your right leg back, and your left leg is bent at a 90-degree angle, making sure your knee and ankle are aligned. Your right leg is as firm and extended as you can get it. Hold for three breaths and feel the stretch in the hip flexor.

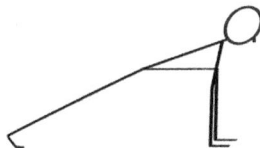

Lunge with a twist - bring your right hand closer to your left foot, circle your left arm up to the ceiling for a twist of the upper body.

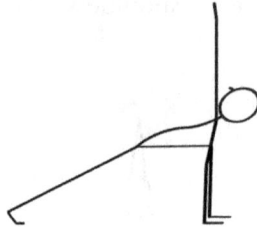

High plank – step your left leg back with your toes on the ground, body parallel with the floor, hands under shoulders, feet hip-width apart, core is tight, and shoulders are rolled back.

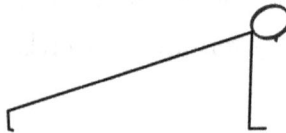

Lower yourself to the ground, leading with the chest and keeping your arms in, close to the body.

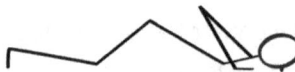

Upward dog - place hands at your sides at chest level with the lower body on the ground; press into your hands and lift upper torso and hips off the ground; arms are straight, rolling the shoulders back and looking back for a slight backbend with the tops of the feet touching the ground.

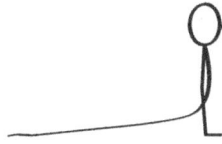

Downward dog – press back onto the balls of the feet, with your feet hip-width apart; place your hands on the ground shoulder-width apart; the body is in a V; press the hips up and press the chest towards the thighs; your head should be between your arms.

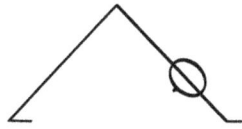

Forward fold – step feet up to hands, reaching your hands towards the floor, and hang forward with a relaxed head.

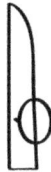

Right runners lunge – place your hands on the ground on either side of your right foot; step left leg back, and right knee is bent at a 90-degree angle, making sure the ankle and knee are aligned. The left leg is as firm and extended as you can get it. Hold for three breaths and feel the stretch in the hip flexor.

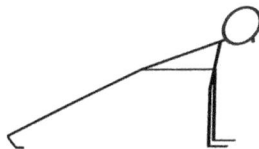

Lunge with a twist - bring your left hand closer to your right foot and circle the right arm towards the ceiling for an upper body twist.

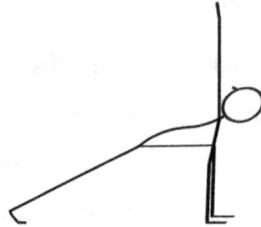

High plank – step your right foot back with toes on the ground, body parallel with the floor, hands under shoulders, feet hip-width apart, core is tight, and shoulders are rolled back.

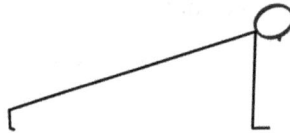

Lower yourself to the ground, leading with the chest and keeping your arms in, close to the body.

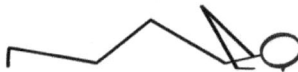

Upward dog - place hands at your sides at chest level with the lower body on the ground; press into your hands and lift upper torso and hips off the ground; arms are straight, rolling the shoulders back and looking back for a slight backbend with the tops of the feet touching the ground.

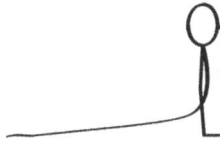

Downward dog – press back onto the balls of your feet, with your feet hip-width apart; hands on the ground shoulder-width apart; the body is in a V; press the hips up and press the chest towards the thighs; your head should be between your arms.

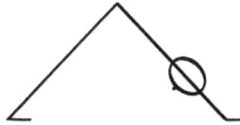

Child's pose - sit with your buttocks on your heels and place your arms straight out in front of you, reaching on the floor, as your forehead touches the ground. This is an active resting pose.

Side Opener – in a child's pose, walk your hands to the right as far as you can, and hold for five seconds to stretch the left side body.

Side Opener – next, walk your hands to the left as far as you can go, and hold for five seconds to stretch the right side body.

Child's pose - sit with your buttocks on your heels and place your arms straight out in front of you, reaching your hands out on the floor, as your forehead touches the ground.

Thread the needle – come into a table-top position with the hands under your shoulders and your knees under your hips. Place your right arm under your left, reaching the shoulder and the ear down to the floor for an upper back and shoulder stretch.

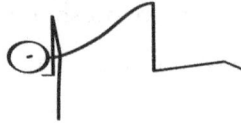

Child's pose - sit with your buttocks on your heels and place your arms straight out in front of you, reaching your hands on the floor, as your forehead touches the ground.

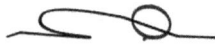

Thread the needle – come into a table-top position with the hands under your shoulders and your knees under your hips. Place your left arm under your right, reaching the shoulder and the ear down to the floor for an extra shoulder stretch.

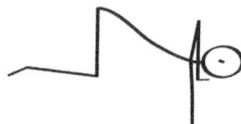

Tip of the day: Stop and take five breaths when you feel stressed. Inhale for four seconds, pause, and extend your exhale for longer. Do this any time you feel stressed, overwhelmed, or not focused.

Focus of the day: Start becoming aware of your breathing when playing your sport. Your breath is your anchor and will always bring you back to a place of stability if you allow it. Practice the 4-7-8 breathing technique to reduce anxiety and help control anger responses (Fletcher, 2019). The 4-7-8 breathing technique is also known as the "relaxing breath". It involves breathing in for four seconds, holding the breath for seven seconds, and exhaling for eight seconds through the mouth. It has been known to slow the heart rate down and slow the central nervous system down as well. If you cannot do the hold for seven and exhale for eight, that is fine. The most important thing is to elongate the exhale as much as you can.

Mindfulness Practice: Becoming Aware of All Parts of the Breath

Sit in a comfortable position. Bring your attention and focus to your breathing. Breathe, and know that you are breathing. Follow your inhalations and your exhalations. Say to yourself, **"breathing in"** when you inhale, and **"breathing out"** when you exhale.

See if you can notice all parts of the breath. Notice where you feel the breath the most. Can you feel the breath coming in and out of your nose? Can you notice your chest rise and fall as you breathe? Can you notice your abdomen rise and fall as you breathe? Pick one of these three places where it is most natural for you to follow your breathing.

See if you can bring your attention to the pause between your breaths. Notice if they are short or long pauses.

Can you notice how each breath is different from the one before? Some inhalations are shorter, and some are longer. Some exhalations are shorter, and some are longer. See if you can notice this difference.

Can you notice that the air you are breathing in is slightly cooler than the air you are breathing out?

Notice any urges you might have to want to stop, to want to think about something. Don't judge, just notice.

Just note these urges and come back to your breathing. As you continue breathing naturally, say to yourself, "breathing in relaxation and calm, breathing out tension and stress." Continue repeating this as you breathe easily.

If your mind wanders and you begin thinking of something, please know that this is natural and normal. As soon as you notice that your mind has wandered, you are practicing mindfulness.

Bring your attention back to your breathing. Continue with this focus for a minute or two.

When you are ready, you may open your eyes.

Lesson Two

Yoga

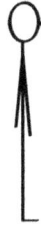

Standing position with eyes closed – feet hip-width apart and arms by your sides. Take a moment to feel your whole body. Take a few breaths, allowing yourself to begin to relax and prepare for slowing down. Notice what it feels like to stand with the eyes closed and be in stillness. Is this difficult or easy? Do you notice any areas of tension in your body? If you do, you can use your breath to focus and send your breathing to those areas. Is your body warm or cool? Can you feel the weight of your body on the floor? Can you feel your feet? Can you feel your breath? Just notice. Now, slowly open your eyes.

Sequence One

Hands at heart -place palms together at chest level.

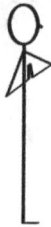

Mountain – circle the arms up, stand tall with the arms overhead parallel to the ears, shoulders relaxed and away from the ears, and feet hip width apart. Take two breaths here.

Baby back bend - lean back slightly and look up, pressing the hips forward.

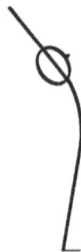

Forward hang – bend at the waist with the hands reaching towards the ground; relax the head and neck; shake the head, yes and no to release the neck.

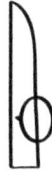

Half lift – inhale, as you slide your hands along your shins, with a straight back, and your shoulders rolled back. Notice your hamstrings and low back in this posture.

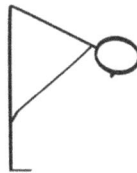

Forward hang – exhale, as you bend from the waist, reaching your hands towards the ground, and hang forward with a relaxed head.

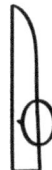

Downward dog – place hands on the ground shoulder-width apart; step your feet back hip-width apart; the body is in a V; press the hips up and press the chest towards the thighs; your head should be between your arms. Can you notice how the body feels in this position?

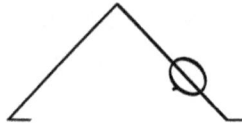

Walk the dog - pedal your heels right and left and focus your attention on your calves.

High plank – bring the body parallel with the floor with the toes on the ground, hands under shoulders, feet hip-width apart, core is tight, and shoulders are rolled back. Hold for a moment and focus on your strength while breathing.

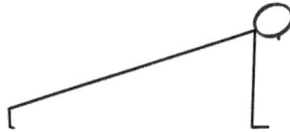

Lower yourself to the ground, leading with the chest and keeping your arms in, close to the body.

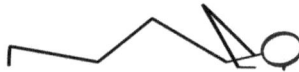

Upward dog - place hands at your sides at chest level with the lower body on the ground; press into your hands and lift upper torso and hips off the ground; arms are straight, rolling shoulders back and looking back for a slight backbend with the tops of the feet touching the ground.

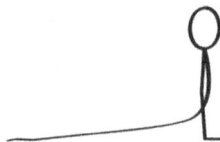

Downward dog – press back on the balls of your feet, with your feet hip-width apart; hands on the ground shoulder-width apart; the body is in a V; press the hips up and press the chest towards the thighs; your head should be between your arms.

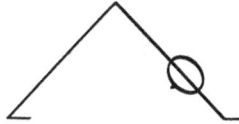

Forward hang - step feet up to your hands for a forward hang, releasing the head and neck, and reaching the hands towards the ground.

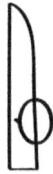

Half lift – inhale, as you slide your hands along your shins with a straight back, upper torso parallel with the floor, and your shoulders are rolled back.

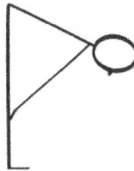

Forward fold – exhale, bend at the waist, reaching arms towards the floor, and hang forward with a relaxed head.

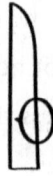

Mountain – inhale as you circle your arms up, standing tall with your arms overhead parallel to your ears, and your shoulders are relaxed.

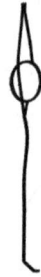

Sequence Two

Hands at heart – place palms together at chest level.

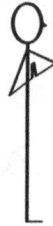

Mountain – circle arms up, standing tall with your arms overhead parallel to your ears, shoulders are relaxed and away from your ears, and feet hip-width apart; take two breaths here.

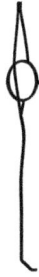

Baby backbend - lean back slightly and look up, pressing hips forward.

Forward hang – bend at the waist, reaching your arms towards the ground and relax your head; shake your head, yes and no to release the neck.

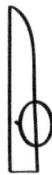

Half lift – inhale, as you slide your hands along your shins with a straight back, and upper torso parallel with the floor; notice your hamstrings and low back in this posture.

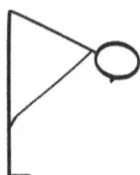

Forward hang – exhale, and bend at the waist, reaching your arms towards the ground; hang forward with a relaxed head.

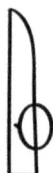

Low runner's lunge – place your hands on the ground on either side of your left foot. Step your right leg back and drop your right leg to the floor, resting the knee and top of the foot on the ground. Keep the left leg bent at a 90-degree angle with the knee and ankle aligned; allow your right hip to sink towards the ground for a hip opener. Next, walk your hands to the inside of your left foot and hold for three breaths. Place your hands back on either side of your left foot.

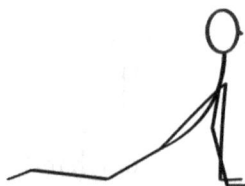

High plank – step your left leg back to meet the right, with the toes on the ground, body parallel to the floor, hands under shoulders, feet hip-width apart, core is tight, and shoulders are rolled back.

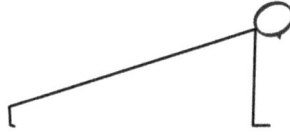

Lower yourself to the ground, leading with the chest and keeping your arms in, close to the body.

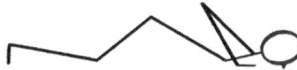

Upward dog - place hands at your sides at chest level with the lower body on the ground; press into your hands and lift upper torso and hips off the ground; arms are straight, rolling shoulders back and looking back for a slight backbend with the tops of the feet touching the ground.

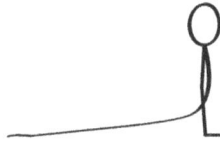

Downward dog – press back onto the balls of the feet, with the feet hip-width apart; hands on the ground shoulder-width apart; the body is in a V; press the hips up and press the chest towards the thighs; your head should be between your arms.

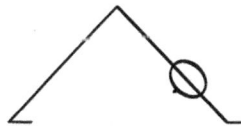

Low runner's lunge- step your right leg forward, bending at a 90-degree angle, with the knee and ankle aligned. Hands are on either side of your foot. Your left leg is back. Now, let your left leg drop to the floor, resting the knee and the top of the foot on the ground. Allow your left hip to sink towards the ground for a hip opener. Next, walk your hands to the inside of your right foot and hold for three breaths. Place your hands back on either side of your foot.

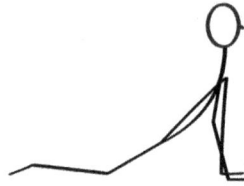

High plank – step your right leg back to meet your left with toes on the ground, body parallel to the floor, hands under shoulders, feet hip-width apart, core is tight, and shoulders are rolled back.

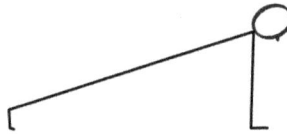

Lower yourself to the ground, leading with the chest and keeping your arms in, close to the body.

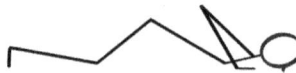

Upward dog - place hands at your sides at chest level with the lower body on the ground; press into your hands and lift upper torso and hips off the ground; arms are straight, rolling the shoulders back and looking back for a slight backbend with the tops of the feet on the floor.

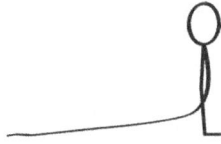

Child's pose - sit with your buttocks on your heels and place your arms straight out in front of you, reaching your hands on the floor, as your forehead touches the ground. Take three breaths here.

Sequence Three

Right pigeon – sit on your right buttocks with your foot close to your groin. Your left leg is extended long behind you with the top of the foot resting on the floor. Make sure your hips are square and facing forward, and your hands are flat on the floor in front of you. Sit up tall first, and then try to walk your hands out in front of you on the floor, reaching with the fingers. This is a hip opener. You may rest your forehead down on the floor if you can.

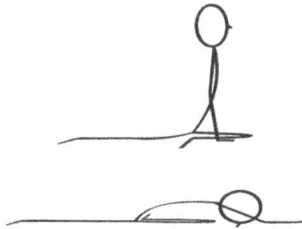

Quad Stretch - sit up, reach around to grab your left foot with your left hand, and press your heel to your butt for a quad stretch. Try to face forward when you do this.

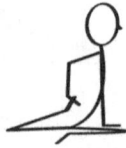

Spinal twist - take your left leg, swing around and place left foot flat on the floor by the outside of your right thigh; inhale, and as you exhale, hug your left knee into your chest and twist your body to the left.

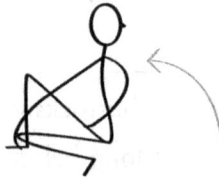

Reclined pigeon (figure four while seated) -take the left ankle and place it on the right knee. Bend right leg with foot flat on the floor. Place your hands behind you under your shoulders, with your fingers facing your feet. Sit up tall with your chest lifted, and press your right thigh against your left ankle to stretch the buttocks.

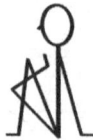

Hamstring stretch - straighten the right leg out in front of you with your toes facing up. Keep the left ankle on the right knee. Inhale, as you reach your arms up, exhale, as you reach forward with your hands towards your right foot.

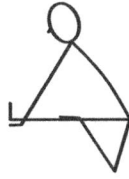

Repeat sequence on the left side (Follow below)

Left pigeon – sit on your left buttocks with your foot close to your groin. Your right leg is extended long behind you, with the top of the foot resting on the floor. Make sure your hips are square and facing forward, and your hands are flat on the floor in front of you. Sit up tall first, and then try to walk your hands on the floor in front of you, reaching with the fingers. This is a hip opener. You may rest your forehead down on the floor if you can.

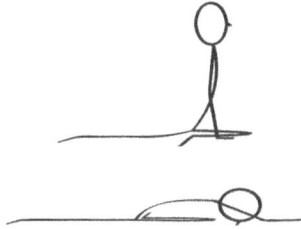

Quad Stretch - sit up, reach around to grab your right foot with your right hand, and press your heel to your butt for a quad stretch.

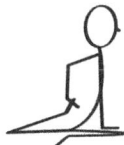

Spinal twist - take your right leg, swing around and place right foot flat on the floor by the outside of your left thigh; inhale, and as you exhale, hug your right knee into your chest and twist your body to the right.

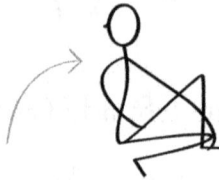

Reclined pigeon (figure four while seated) -take the right ankle and place it on the left knee. Bend the left leg with foot flat on the floor. Place your hands behind you with your fingers facing your feet. Sit up tall with your chest lifted, and press your left thigh against your right ankle to stretch the buttocks.

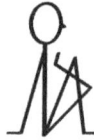

Hamstring stretch - straighten the left leg out in front of you with the toes pointed up. Keep the right ankle on the left knee. Inhale, as you reach your arms up, exhale, as you reach forward with your hands towards your left foot.

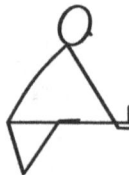

Tip of the day: Practice a body scan at any time during your day when you need to settle in. This can also be used before bed if you have trouble falling asleep.

Focus of the day: Check in with the body! Paying attention to the body and becoming aware of the body is extremely important to an athlete, to be able to sense your body's position and form, your ability for accurate movement, and your balance. This heightened awareness of body sensations allows you to make adjustments in shifting your weight, using your strength and power, and working on precise timing. According to Saltzman (2018), it can also help you know whether you are training too much or training too little. Awareness can also help you distinguish between fatigue that is typical for your body and deep exhaustion that can lead to more serious signs of injury. Over time, as you become more aware of your body's sensations, you will begin to realize that sensations are temporary (they come and go), but pain persists and lasts longer!

Mindfulness Practice: Becoming Aware of the Body

I'd like you to get comfortable by lying down. Take a few deep breaths, in through the nose and out through the nose. Visualize your inhalations, expanding from deep within the belly, extending up to the rib cage, and making your way to your chest. Allow each exhale to be smooth and soft. Continue to breathe like this for a couple of breaths.

Allow everything to go; any responsibilities, things to do, any type of work. You are letting it all go…

We will now begin the body scan exercise. I'd like you to start by focusing on your toes. See if you can feel your toes, noticing any sensations such as warmth, coolness, tightness, or softness. Just bring all your awareness to how your toes feel, and if you feel nothing, that is fine as well. Now, relax and soften your ankles, calf muscles, knees, and thigh muscles. See if you can notice any sensations in these areas, allowing these body parts to soften, release, and relax. If you find you are lost in thought, imagine a beautiful sunny sky with some white, fluffy clouds. Imagine that each thought floats away on a cloud in the sky, and then bring yourself back to your body scan.

Now, relax and soften the backs of your legs, buttocks, and your pelvic area. From your hips down to your toes, your entire lower body should be relaxed and soft.

Now, focus on your belly, softening and releasing any tension here, and imagining that your tummy is empty and relaxed. Work your way up to the chest and let go of tension or tightness here as well. Let's bring your focus to your back. Breathe deeply in, and as you breathe out, slowly relax and release any tension you may have in your back, starting from your lower back, moving your way up to the upper back. Now, bring your attention to your shoulders. Lift them up to your ears and then release them completely, allowing them to melt into the floor.

Bring your attention to your upper arms, elbows, lower arms, and both hands. Relax, soften, and loosen both arms and hands. Now it is time to relax your neck and jaw muscles. Take a deep breath in, and as you breathe out, let go of any tension you may be holding in your neck and jaw.

Focus on your face, making sure to soften the mouth, cheeks, nose, eyes, and eyebrows. Finally, bring your awareness to the top of your head.

Now, try to feel your entire body lying on the surface you are on. Try to feel complete relaxation, calmness, and peacefulness throughout your entire being.

Take a few more deep breaths and enjoy this feeling of relaxation and calm for a little while longer. I'd like you to now slowly bring your attention back to the room.

Begin noticing the sounds around you, and when you're ready, open your eyes.

LESSON THREE

Yoga

Sequence One

Hands at heart – place palms together at chest level.

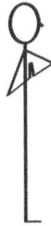

Mountain – circle the arms up and stand tall with the feet hip-width apart, the arms overhead parallel to the ears, and the shoulders are relaxed.

Half-moon to the right - stand with the knees and feet together, arms overhead, interlacing your fingers, with your pointer fingers facing up.

Inhale, as you reach up, exhale, as you reach your arms to the right. Keep chest and chin up, squeeze your inner thighs together to open the left side.

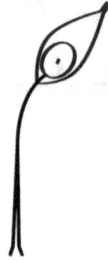

Half-moon to the left - stand with knees and feet together, arms overhead, interlacing your fingers with the pointer fingers reaching up. Inhale, as you reach up, exhale, as you reach your arms to the left. Keep chest and chin up, squeeze your inner thighs together to open the right side.

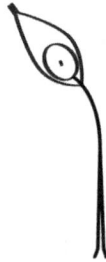

Baby backbend - lean back slightly and look up, pressing hips forward.

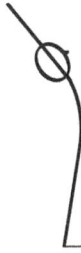

Forward hang - bend at the waist, reaching the arms towards the floor, and hang forward with a relaxed head.

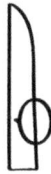

Half lift – inhale, as you slide your hands along your shins with a straight back, upper torso lifting parallel to the ground.

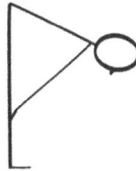

Forward fold – exhale, as you bend at the waist, reaching your hands to the floor. Hang forward with a relaxed head.

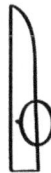

High plank – step legs back with your toes on the ground, hands under shoulders, feet hip-width apart, core is tight, and shoulders are rolled back.

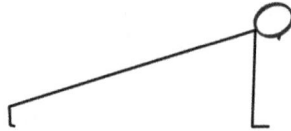

Downward dog - press back to the balls of the feet, hands on the ground shoulder-width apart; the body is in a V; press the hips up and press the chest towards the thighs; your head should be between your arms.

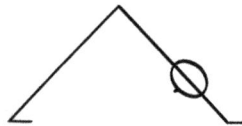

Downward dog to high plank - continue to move from downward dog to high plank (inhale to plank and exhale to downward dog). Repeat these five times.

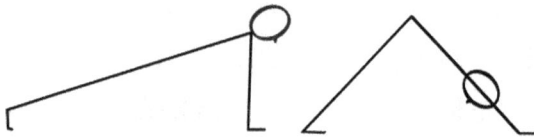

Child's pose – sit with buttocks on the heels, reach arms out in front of you, check-in with the mind, breathe in relaxation and breathe out tension.

Low lunge – bring your right leg forward at a 90-degree angle with the knee over the ankle. The left leg rests on the ground, with the knee and the top of the foot resting on the floor. Press your left hip into the floor for a hip flexor stretch.

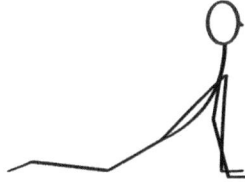

Lizard pose (low lunge forearm stretch) - place hands to the inside of the right foot, and try to lower your forearms down to the ground if you can. Let the right leg fan out to the side.

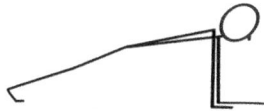

High plank – step right leg back with toes on the ground, hands under shoulders, feet hip-width apart, core is tight, and shoulders are rolled back.

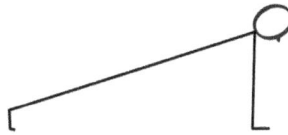

Lower yourself to the ground, leading with the chest and keeping your arms in, close to the body.

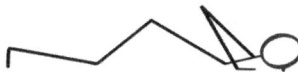

Upward dog - place hands at your sides at chest level with the lower body on the ground; press into your hands and lift upper torso and hips off the ground; arms are straight, rolling shoulders back and looking back for a slight backbend with the tops of the feet on the floor.

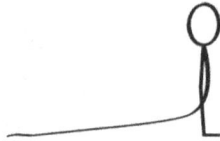

Downward dog – press back onto the balls of your feet, with your feet hip-width apart; hands on the ground shoulder-width apart; the body is in a V; press the hips up and press the chest towards the thighs; your head should be between your arms.

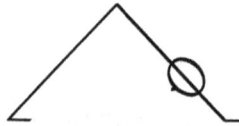

Low lunge – step the left leg forward at a 90-degree angle with the knee over the ankle, and let the right leg rest on the floor, with the knee and the top of the foot resting on the ground. Hands on either side of your left foot. Press your right hip towards the floor for a hip flexor stretch.

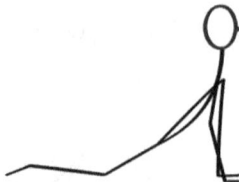

Lizard pose (low lunge forearm stretch) – place your hands to the inside of the left foot, and bring your forearms to the ground if you can. Let the left leg fan out to the left side.

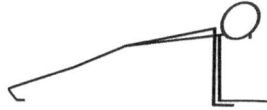

High Plank – step the left leg back with the toes on the ground, hands under shoulders, feet hip-width apart, core is tight, and shoulders are rolled back.

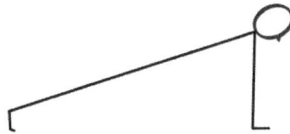

Lower yourself to the ground, leading with the chest and keeping your arms in, close to the body.

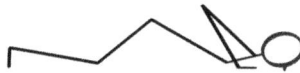

Upward dog - place hands at your sides at chest level with the lower body on the ground; press into your hands and lift upper torso and hips off the ground; arms are straight, rolling shoulders back and looking back for a slight backbend with the tops of the feet on the ground.

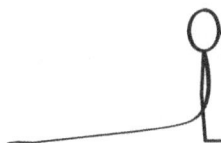

Child's pose - sit with your buttocks on your heels and place your arms straight out in front of you, reaching your hands on the floor, as your forehead touches the ground. Take three breaths here and relax.

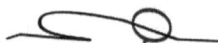

Sequence Two

Table-top – position yourself on the floor on your hands and knees, with your knees under your hips, and your hands under your shoulders.

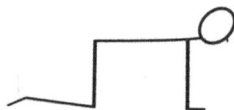

Cat Cow - inhale to cow, by dropping the belly and lifting the chin. Exhale to cat, by rounding the back and bringing your chin to your chest. Repeat five times.

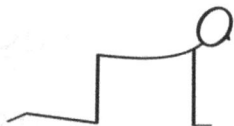

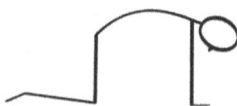

Spinal balance – on all fours, lift the right arm straight out in front and lift the left leg straight behind, reaching with the fingers and toes. Both should be parallel with the ground. Hold for five seconds. Return to table-top.

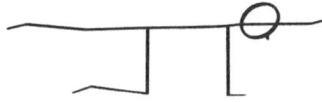

Spinal balance - lift the left arm straight out in front and lift the right leg straight behind. Both should be parallel with the ground. Reach with the fingers and point the toes. Hold for five seconds. Return to table-top.

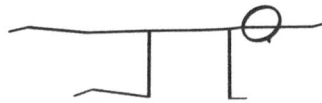

Repeat spinal balance two more times on each side.

Bird-dog – in table-top position, lift your right arm and left leg straight. Move the right elbow in and the left knee in to meet and hold. Repeat five times slowly.

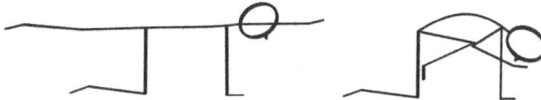

Bird-dog - lift your left arm and right leg straight. Move the left elbow in and right knee in to meet and hold. Repeat five times slowly.

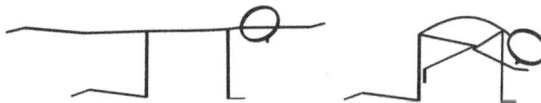

Single bow pose - lift the right arm and left leg, bend the left leg and reach around to grab the ankle with your right hand. Kick your left foot into your hand for a full stretch. Hold for five seconds.

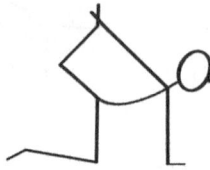

Single bow pose – lift the left arm and right leg, bend the right leg and reach around to grab the ankle with your left hand. Kick your right foot into your hand for a full stretch. Hold for five seconds.

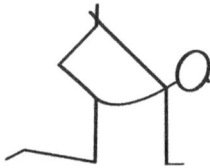

Forearm stretches - in a tabletop position, turn your hands around so that your fingers are facing your feet. Gently move back and forth to stretch the forearms or move in circles if you wish.

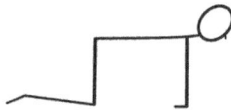

Sequence Three

Butterfly stretch – in a seated position bring the soles of the feet together. Try to lean forward as much as you can, reaching your arms forward for an inner thigh stretch.

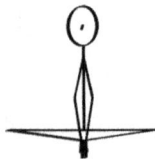

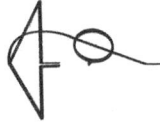

Pike stretch – both legs are straight out in front of you. Inhale, and reach arms up, exhale, as you reach your hands for your feet for a hamstring stretch. Try lifting your heels off the ground and reach for your feet for an extra calf stretch. Hold for five seconds.

Flow in a pike position – inhale, and reach arms up above your head, and exhale as you reach forward to pike. Repeat this sequence five times.

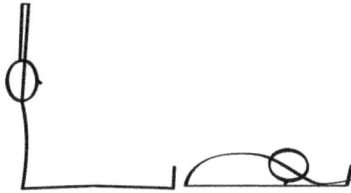

Seated pike position – with legs straight out in front of you, place your hands behind your head and gently press on the back of the head as you lean your body forward (this is a great upper back and neck stretch). Hold for five seconds. Repeat three times.

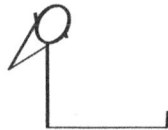

Tip of the day: Finger Touching Mantra (Biegel & Corbin, 2018) - Hold out one hand and touch your thumb to each finger, starting with the pinky, ring finger, middle finger, and pointer finger. As you touch each finger, you say a mantra that will help you. For instance, here are some popular mantras that people use to help them relax, calm down, and reduce anxiety.

I am so calm

I can do this

I will get through

You repeat this mantra as many times as you need in order to feel better. Let's practice now.

Focus of the day: You are in control of your mind! No one else is. As Burdick (2014) points out, you need to start learning to flip the switch or change the channel when you are in a bad place swirling with negativity about yourself. You must learn to separate the person from the performance. Your performance does not define you! You are not your thoughts!!! They are just opinions and ideas you have as a result of thinking. They are not truths. Start saying to yourself that, "I am having the thought that"… Instead of believing it! Think of witnessing your thoughts and letting them go.

Mindfulness: Becoming Aware of Thoughts and the Mind

Let's find a comfortable position and settle in. Bring your attention to your breathing. You are breathing naturally and normally and tuning in to where you feel your breath the most right now. Following each inhale and exhale as best as you can, saying to yourself, breathing in and breathing out. Let's follow a few breaths like that, so we begin to settle ourselves.

Now, we will begin exploring and working with our thoughts. We are not trying to stop thinking, because that is impossible. The goal of this practice is to bring awareness to the fact that we are thinking and then take note.

So, let's begin by imagining a beautiful stream of flowing water. This can be a stream you know or a stream you are imagining in your mind. Take a moment to visualize the beautiful stream now. Picture the details of this scene. Imagine hearing the sounds of the water, imagine visualizing what type of day it is, sunny, cloudy, blue sky. Imagine the trees that are nearby and the flowers that are blooming all around you. Imagine all the details, and then picture yourself sitting near this stream. Imagine that leaves are floating by in the stream. Watch the leaves float away, passing you by. All of the beautiful colors of the fall leaves float gently down the stream.

In order to become aware of your thoughts, you will let your mind go, and every time you have a thought, note it **"thinking"**, and then see if you can imagine each of your thoughts being placed on a leaf and floating down the stream. Try to be an observer from the outside, like watching a movie of your thoughts. Let them come, and let them go, placing them on the leaves, and watching them float away. Any thought that pops into your mind, you will imagine putting it on a leaf, and watching it float away. Even if the thought is positive, place it on the leaf, and watch it float away. You might think to yourself at some point that this is stupid, or you can't wait until this is over. Just place that thought on a leaf, and watch it float down the stream. If you do not have any thoughts at all, just picture your stream flowing as you sit right on the bank, watching. Another thought will eventually pop into your head for you to place on a leaf in the stream. (Pause for 1 minute). Let's take one last moment to visualize this stream with the water running and the leaves being carried by the water. Now, let's slowly bring your focus back to the fact that you are breathing. Take a nice big inhale through the nose and exhale through the nose, and slowly open your eyes.

LESSON FOUR

Yoga

Sequence One

Neck stretches right – in a seated position, bring your right ear to your right shoulder and hold for five seconds. Repeat five times.

Neck stretches left – in a seated position bring your left ear to your left shoulder and hold for five seconds. Repeat five times.

Neck turns - turn your head as far as you can to the right side and then as far as you can to the left side. Repeat five times.

Neck rolls – bring your chin to your chest, then roll your head to the right, bringing your right ear to your right shoulder. Hold for five seconds. Then, roll your head forward and to the left, bringing your left ear to your left shoulder. Hold for five seconds. Repeat four times on each side.

Side stretch to the right – with your legs crossed, lift your left arm up overhead and then lean to the right side with your right hand on the ground for a left side opener.

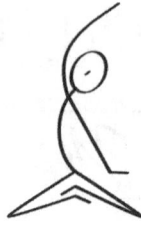

Side stretch to the left – with your legs crossed, lift your right arm up overhead and then lean to the left side with your left hand on the ground for a right side opener.

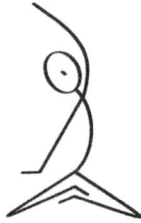

Repeat side stretches six times total, moving back and forth from right to left.

Seated mountain twist – inhale, as you lift arms up parallel to the ears, and exhale, as you twist your upper body to the right side, placing your right hand on the ground behind you and your left hand on the ground in front of you.

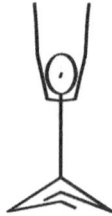

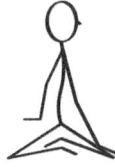

Seated mountain twist – inhale, as you lift arms up parallel to the ears, and exhale, as you twist your upper body to the left side, placing your left hand on the ground behind you and your right hand on the ground in front of you.

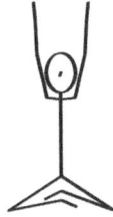

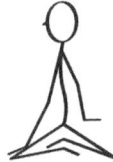

Repeat mountain twists six times total moving back and forth from right to left side.

Reverse table - in a seated position with hands flat on the ground behind you under your shoulders, and feet hip-width apart, press up into your hands and feet as you lift your hips off the ground, roll your shoulders back and open your chest. Hold for five seconds.

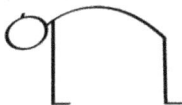

Eagle arm stretch right – in a seated position, bring your arms straight out in front of you. Cross your right arm over left arm, bend at the elbows, hands are back to back or palms touching, press arms away from the body for an upper back stretch. Begin to move arms up, lifting chin, and down with chin to the chest. Move up and down in this position four times.

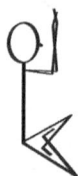

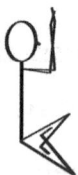

Eagle arm stretch left – in a seated position, bring your arms straight out in front of you. Cross your left arm over your right arm, bend at the elbows, hands are back to back or palms touching, press arms away from the body for an upper back stretch. Begin to move arms up, lifting chin, and down with chin to the chest. Move up and down in this position four times.

Reverse table - in a seated position with hands flat on the floor behind you under your shoulders, and feet hip-width apart, press up into your hands and feet as you lift your hips off the ground, roll your shoulders back and open your chest. Hold for five seconds.

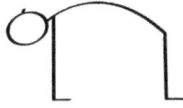

Butterfly stretch - in a seated position, bring the soles of the feet together. Try to lean forward as much as you can, reaching your hands towards the floor for an inner thigh stretch.

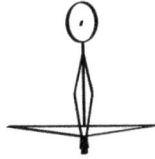

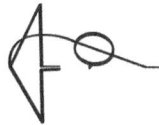

Straddle – separate your legs out as wide as you can in a seated position. Inhale, reach up, and then exhale as you reach forward, with your hands as far as you can.

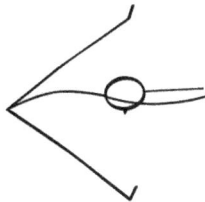

Sequence Two

Table-top – position yourself on the floor, on your hands and knees, with your knees under your hips, and your hands under your shoulders.

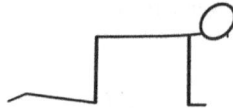

Cat cow - inhale to cow, by dropping the belly and lifting the chin. Exhale to cat, by rounding the back and bringing your chin to your chest. Repeat five times.

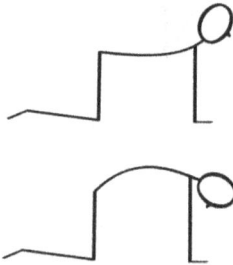

Spinal balance - lift the right arm straight out in front, and lift the left leg straight behind, reaching with the fingers and pointing the toes. Both should be parallel with the ground. Hold for five seconds.

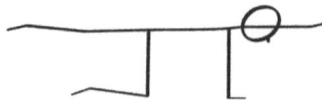

Spinal balance – lift the left arm straight out in front, and lift the right leg straight behind, reaching with the fingers and pointing the toes. Both should be parallel with the ground. Hold for five seconds.

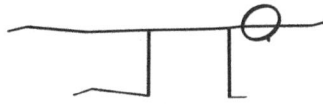

Single bow pose - lift the right arm and left leg, bend the left leg and reach around to grab the ankle with your right hand. Press your left foot into your hand for a full stretch.

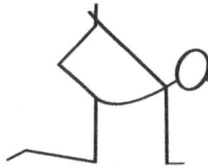

Single bow pose – lift the left arm forward and right leg back, bend right leg, reach around to grab the ankle with your left hand. Press your right foot into your hand and roll your shoulders back.

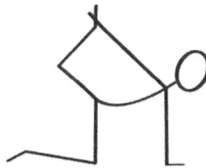

Camel on knees – place your shins on the floor, and make sure your knees are under your hips, hands on your low back, press hips forward, and then reach one hand at a time back to your ankles if you can. Continue to press hips forward, and let head hang back for a mini backbend if you can.

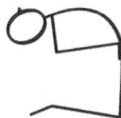

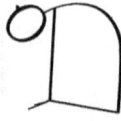

Child's pose - sit back on your heels and place your arms straight out in front of you, reaching on the floor, as your forehead touches the ground for a counter stretch.

Frog pose - start on all fours in table-top position, widen the distance between the knees as much as you can without straining, bring your forearms to the ground, and breathe for an inner thigh stretch.

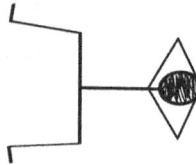

Hero pose - sit on the ground with your buttocks between your legs. Your feet are on each side of your buttocks. This is to stretch the quads, so when you are ready, you can begin to lean back as far as you can on your elbows or lay all the way down if you can.

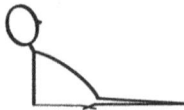

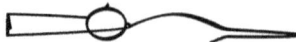

Sequence Three

Scorpion pose right- laying on the stomach with arms out like a T, bend right leg, reach it up towards the ceiling, and then allow the leg to fall all the way to the ground to the left side with your hip coming off the ground.

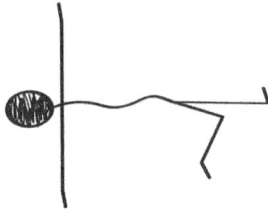

Scorpion pose left- laying on the stomach with arms out like a T, bend left leg, reach it up towards the ceiling, and then allow the leg to fall all the way to the ground to the right side with your hip coming off the ground.

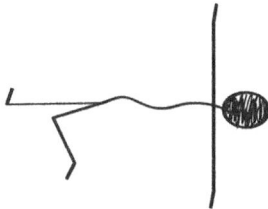

Bow pose - bend both legs, reach around for your ankles, flex your feet, and press your feet into your hands, lifting your chest and shoulders off the ground.

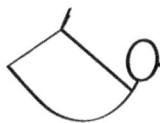

Windshield wipers – on your stomach, bend your knees, and sway legs from side to side, head resting on your hands for a low back massage and opener. Keep your torso and shoulders flat on the ground.

Child's pose - sit back with your buttocks on your heels and place your arms straight out in front of you, reaching on the floor, as your forehead touches the ground. Take three breaths here and relax.

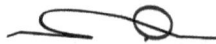

Puppy pose – come into a table-top position, with your knees under hips, and hands under your shoulders. Start leaning your buttocks towards your heels and reach your arms forward on the ground, without allowing the belly to rest on the thighs. You may rest your forehead on the ground.

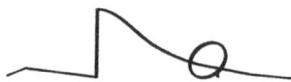

Tip of the day: Five Senses for Anxiety to Stay in the Moment: This is a coping technique for anxiety. If you ever feel overwhelmed and completely anxiety-ridden, you should try this exercise. You immediately stop what you're doing and notice five things that you can see, four things you can feel (these can be physical sensations or emotions), three things you can hear, two things you can smell, and one thing you can taste. This helps with anxiety and stress by bringing you back to reality (Mayo Clinic, 2020).

Focus of the day: 90 Second Rule! Response vs. Reaction. An emotion only physically stays with us for 90 seconds because there is a chemical process that occurs! After 90 seconds, if we still feel an emotion, it is because we are fueling the emotion with our thoughts and images. Sadness is the only exception to this. It can last for up to 72 hours. During your sport, when you get angry, stop and allow 90 seconds to go by before reacting (Stone, 2019).

Start paying attention to your body when you experience emotions. Your body will hold your emotions in certain areas. If you can become aware of what you are feeling in your body and what you are thinking in your mind when you feel anger or frustration, you give yourself space to respond instead of reacting.

According to Mindful Schools (2015), three things happen when you experience an emotion (positive or negative):

1. You feel sensations in your body

2. You start self-talk & thinking and/or telling stories in your mind

3. You visualize images in your mind

Try to start paying attention to these three things that happen immediately when you experience an emotion, giving you time to respond.

Mindfulness Activity: Learning Your Emotions

I want you to imagine a place that is safe and peaceful for you. It can be anywhere you want in the world. It can be at a beach, or on a mountain, in an open field, or in your home. Picture all the details of this place. Imagine the colors in this place, imagine the sights in this place, and the sounds you may hear. The more detail, the better. Picture yourself in this place, feeling free, light, and relaxed. Enjoy these feelings of peace and calm here. Feel in your body where you notice this relaxing and calm feeling. Perhaps you feel lighter or heavier? Just notice.

Now, we are going to explore some emotions and notice where in your body you sense these emotions. The goal of this practice is to learn where we hold certain emotions in our body so that we can have a greater mind-body connection. Let's start out with the feeling of pride. Think of something you are proud of that you have done lately or maybe someone you are proud of (pause). Notice where you feel this feeling of pride in your body. Next, let's think of the emotion happiness. What makes you genuinely happy when you think about it? Can you remember a time when you felt pure happiness or joy? Now, notice where you feel this in your body.

Now, let's think of the feeling sadness. Has there been a time when you have felt sad? Think back to this time and notice where in your body you feel sadness.

Let's think of the emotion kindness. Think of how it feels when you do something kind for someone else, or when someone does something kind for you. Let the emotion of kindness spread throughout your body and notice where in your body you feel this emotion.

Now, let's think of the emotion fear. Has there been a time when you felt fear? How does that emotion feel in your body? Do you notice where in the body you can feel fear? Remember, we are just noticing how our physical body responds when we think or feel an emotion. Just sit with that for a moment.

Lastly, let's think of the emotion gratitude. Feel the feelings that arise when you think of being grateful for something or someone in your life. Reflect for a moment on the feeling of gratitude and what you are grateful for in your life right now at this moment. Let that feeling spread throughout your body and notice where you feel this emotion.

When we learn to bring our attention to where in the body we feel emotions, we can learn more about ourselves, particularly noticing when we might be triggered to react a certain way that we may later regret. Making the connection between our emotions and our body sensations is enormously powerful information for us.

Now, let's bring our attention back to our breathing. Please take three deep breaths inhaling through your nose and exhaling through your nose. When you are ready, you can open your eyes.

LESSON FIVE

Yoga

Sequence One

Lay on the back - (Use bands if available)

Rolling hips - bring knees to chest and arms out like a T on the ground. Now, move the knees from right to left at your own pace.

Right hamstring stretch - place your right foot in the band and straighten the leg to the ceiling. Your left leg is straight, resting on the ground. Gently pull your right leg towards you for a hamstring stretch. Hold for ten seconds.

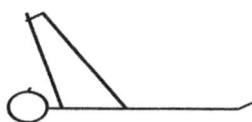

Inner thigh stretch – with the leg straight, move the right leg all the way to the right, hovering off the ground for an inner thigh stretch.

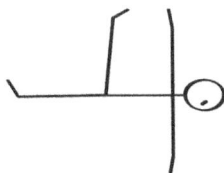

Spinal twist – next, move the right leg all the way to the left side, crossing your body for a spinal twist.

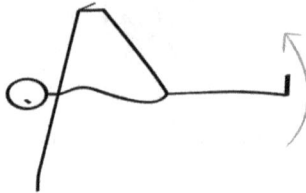

Moving back and forth - continue to move the right leg back and forth at your own pace six times.

Left hamstring stretch - place your left foot in the band and straighten the leg the best you can. The right leg is straight, resting on the ground. Gently pull your left leg towards you for a hamstring stretch. Hold for ten seconds.

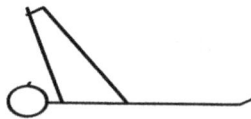

Inner thigh stretch – with the leg straight, move the left leg all the way to the left, hovering off the ground for an inner thigh stretch.

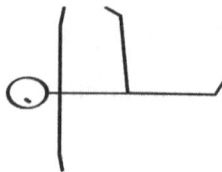

Spinal twist – next, move the left leg across your body to the right for a spinal twist.

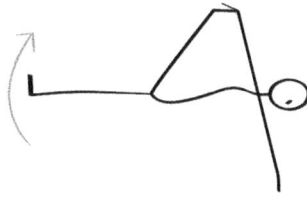

Moving back and forth - continue to move the left leg back and forth at your own pace six times.

Double hamstring stretch - place both legs in the band and straighten them to the ceiling with flexed feet. Hold for ten seconds. Band work is complete.

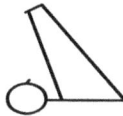

Figure four - lay on your back and put your right ankle on your left knee; grab under your left leg and pull into you.

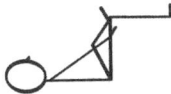

Cross leg stretch - cross right knee over the left knee, and let legs fall to the left for a twist. Turn your head to the right and place your arms out like a T on the ground.

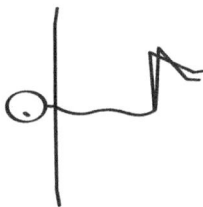

Figure four - lay on back and place the left ankle on right knee; grab under your right leg and pull into you.

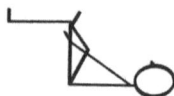

Cross leg stretch - cross left knee over the right knee and let legs fall to the right. Turn your head to the left and place your arms out like a T on the ground.

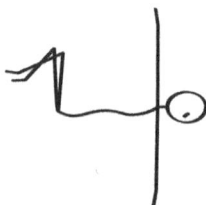

Roll-up - lay on the ground with arms overhead and legs straight on the ground. Inhale, and as you exhale, slowly lift one vertebra at a time off the ground and try to roll up to a pike position, reaching your hands to your feet. Slowly lower back down. Repeat five times slowly. This is a great core exercise.

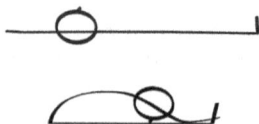

Flowing sequence in pike position – sit in a pike position. Inhale, and lift your arms up, parallel to the ears. Then, exhale to a pike position, reaching your hands to your feet. Repeat five times.

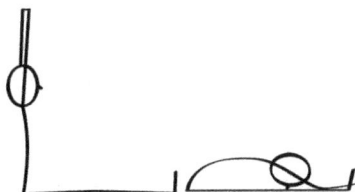

Sequence Two (Balancing in a standing position)

Right side

Tree pose – shift your weight to your left foot and place your right foot either on the lower shin or upper thigh of the left leg; knee is parallel to the ground, and hands come to the heart with the palms together or above your head for a balance. Hold for ten seconds.

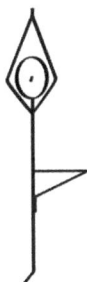

Dancer's Pose – lift your right leg behind you, and with your right hand, grab the top of the foot or ankle. Stretch your left arm up parallel to your ear, and begin to lean forward, pressing your foot into your hand, as you reach out and lower your left arm until it is parallel with the ground. This is a balance pose. Hold for ten seconds.

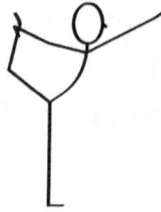

Eagles Pose – shift your weight to the left foot, take your right leg and wrap it over the left knee, with toes pointing down. If you can, wrap the right foot behind the left leg while maintaining balance. Take the right arm and cross over the left arm, bend at the elbows, and hands are back-to-back or palms touching. Bend your left knee at a 90-degree angle. Chest is open, shoulders are away from the ears. Hold for five seconds.

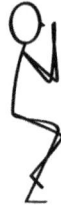

Left Side

Tree pose – shift your weight to your right foot, place your left foot either on the lower shin or upper thigh of the right leg; knee is parallel to the ground, and hands come to the heart with the palms touching or above your head for a balance. Hold for ten seconds.

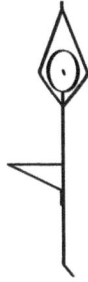

Dancer's Pose – lift your left leg behind you, and with your left hand, grab the top of the foot or the ankle. Stretch your right arm up parallel to your ear, and begin to lean forward, pressing your foot into your hand, as you reach out and lower your right arm until it is parallel with the ground. This is a balance pose. Hold for ten seconds.

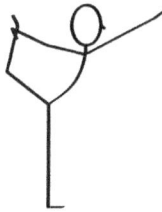

Eagles Pose – shift your weight to your right foot, take left leg and wrap it over the right knee, with the toes pointing down. If you can, wrap the left foot behind the right leg, while maintaining balance. Take the left arm and cross over the right arm, bend at the elbows, and hands are back-to-back or palms touching. Bend your right knee at a 90-degree angle. Chest is open, shoulders are away from the ears. Hold for five seconds.

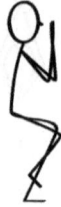

Sequence Three (Standing)

Mountain - stand with the feet hip-width apart. As you inhale, bring your arms overhead parallel to the ears, and shoulders relaxed. Take two breaths here.

Chair – place your knees and feet together, bend your knees and sit back in an imaginary chair, arms are parallel to your ears; tighten the lower body and squeeze your inner thighs together. Weight is on your heels. This is a strengthening exercise for your lower body.

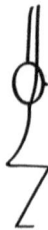

Forward hang - bend at the waist, reaching your hands towards the ground with a relaxed head.

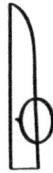

Roll up like a rag doll – slowly begin rolling your body up with the head being the last lifted.

Repeat this sequence ten times: mountain, chair, forward hang, roll up like a rag doll

Tip of the day: When you are stressed, start noticing what is going on in your body, and what begins to happen emotionally. See if you can notice where in your body you feel stress.

Focus of the day: Biegel and Corbin (2018) talk about knowing your stressors so that you can start to recognize and reduce your stress. Effective stress management starts with identifying your sources of stress and developing strategies to manage them. One way to do this is to make a list of the situations, concerns, or challenges that trigger your stress. Take a moment to write down some of the top issues you're facing right now. You'll notice that some of your stressors are events that happen to you, while others seem to originate within you (negative self-talk, expectations you put on yourself).

Mindfulness Activity: Remembering A Time of Wellness (Burdick, 2014)

Heart and Belly Breathing (Harper et al., 2017)

Place one hand on your heart and one hand on your belly. Continue to breathe naturally and normally with your hands in these places and notice the pace of your breathing. See if you can tune into how slowly or rapidly you are breathing. See if you can feel your chest rise and fall as you breathe. See if you can feel your belly rise and fall as you breathe. Try to follow each inhale and exhale as you breathe with complete peace, relaxation, and a sense of calm. There is nothing else you need to be doing right now other than trying to follow your breath. (Allow another minute of this breathing).

Now, if you would like to find a position lying down that would be more comfortable, please get into that position. We will now try to remember a time when you felt great, both physically and mentally. A time when physically, you felt you were at your best; you felt healthy, strong, and in good shape. During this time, you also felt really happy. You were in a good place mentally, and you were very excited about where you were in life at that point. I'll give you a moment to recall such a time when you felt on top of the world.

If you are having trouble finding a time that you felt this awesome, I would ask you to imagine what it would look like for you to be in your best health both mentally and physically.

Remember the details of this time. How old were you? What did you look like then? Were there any changes from now? Imagine what you were doing? Who were you with? Just breathe in, and allow this memory to grow and expand in your mind. Remember why you felt so good and happy with your life. What was going on at that time? Take a moment to reminisce or use your imagination to picture this time of optimal health. Who were the people in your life at that time that mattered most to you? Remember how those people made you feel. Recall how nice it was to feel so proud, excited, happy, confident, and secure. See if you could really tune into those feelings now and allow those feelings to grow inside you at this moment, so that now, you feel strong, confident, fit, secure, proud, happy, and excited in life. Take a moment to feel these wonderful feelings inside.

Now, I want you to imagine that your body is in the best shape right now. Your muscles are strong and flexible. Your endurance is at its best. You are fast and powerful. Imagine your agility and coordination are at the top of your game. Your balance is on point. You feel the best you have ever felt! You are ready to conquer the world and perform at your best. Nothing can stop you! Both physically and mentally, you are where you need and want to be.

Hold on to this feeling for a few more moments and enjoy this optimal health you are experiencing. (Pause for a minute)

When you are ready, take a nice deep breath, in through your nose and out through your nose. You may slowly open your eyes.

LESSON SIX

Yoga

Sequence One

Table-top – take a position on the floor, with your knees under your hips, and your hands under your shoulders.

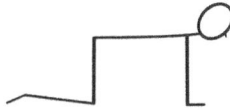

Cat Cow – inhale, belly drops and chin lifts. Exhale, round the back and bring your chin to your chest. Repeat five times.

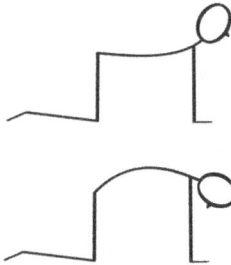

Spinal balance - lift the right arm straight out in front of you and lift the left leg straight behind you; fingers reaching and toes pointing. Both should be parallel with the ground. Hold for five seconds. Come back to table-top position. Repeat this spinal balance hold five times.

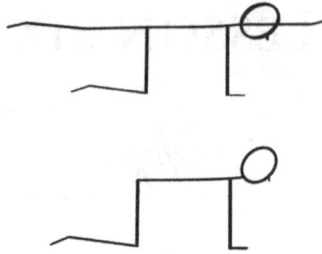

Spinal balance - lift the left arm straight out in front of you and lift the right leg straight behind you; fingers reaching and toes pointing. Both should be parallel with the ground. Hold for five seconds. Come back to table-top position. Repeat this spinal balance five times.

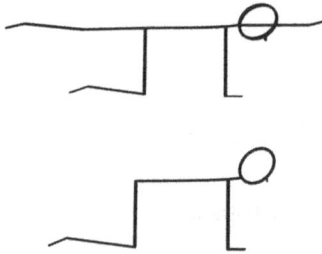

Child's pose - sit with your buttocks on your heels and place your arms straight out in front of you, reaching on the floor, as your forehead touches the ground. Take three breaths here and relax.

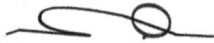

Puppy pose – come into table-top position, with your knees under hips, and hands under shoulders. Start leaning your buttocks towards your heels and reach your arms forward on the ground, without allowing the belly to rest on the thighs. You may rest your forehead on the ground if you can.

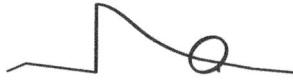

Downward dog – lift the knees off the ground, press back to the balls of the feet; hands on the ground shoulder-width apart; feet are hip-width apart; the body is in a V; press the hips up and press the chest towards the thighs; your head should be between your arms.

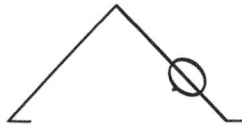

Forward hang – walk feet up to meet hands, reaching your hands towards the ground, relaxing the head and neck.

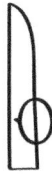

Half lift – inhale, as you slide your hands along your shins with a straight back, upper torso coming up parallel to the ground.

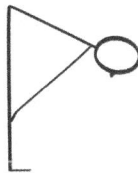

Forward fold – exhale, as you bend at the waist, reaching your hands towards the ground. Hang forward with a relaxed head.

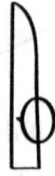

Mountain – inhale, as you stand tall with your arms overhead parallel to your ears, shoulders relaxed and away from your ears.

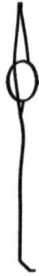

Sequence Two

3 Sun Salutations

Mountain – stand with the feet hip-width apart; inhale, as you reach arms overhead parallel to your ears, shoulders are relaxed and away from the ears.

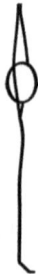

Forward hang – exhale, as you bend at the waist, reaching your hands to the floor. Hang forward with a relaxed head.

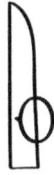

Half lift – inhale, as you slide hands along shins with a straight back, upper torso coming up parallel to the ground.

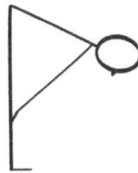

Forward hang – exhale, as you bend at the waist, reaching the hands to the floor. Hang forward with a relaxed head.

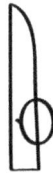

High plank – place hands on the floor shoulder-width apart; step both feet back hip-width apart, core is tight, body parallel to the floor, and shoulders are rolled back.

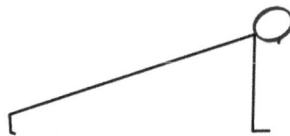

Lower yourself to the ground, leading with the chest and keeping your arms in, close to the body.

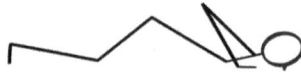

Upward dog - place hands at your sides at chest level with the lower body on the ground; press into your hands and lift upper torso and hips off the ground; arms are straight, rolling the shoulders back and looking back for a slight backbend with the tops of the feet on the ground.

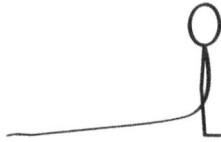

Downward dog – press back to the balls of your feet; hands on the ground shoulder-width apart; feet are hip-width apart; the body is in a V; press the hips up and press the chest towards the thighs; your head should be between your arms.

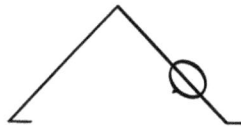

Forward hang – step your feet up to your hands, reaching your hands to the floor, with a relaxed head.

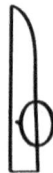

Repeat sequence TWO; sun salutations three more times starting with mountain pose

Sequence Three

Mountain - stand with the feet hip-width apart; inhale, as you reach arms overhead parallel to your ears, shoulders are relaxed and away from the ears.

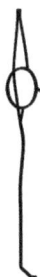

Warrior 1 right side – step your right leg forward with the knee bent at a 90-degree angle, and left leg is straight behind you with your left foot turned out slightly. Square your hips to face forward and reach arms up parallel to your ears. This is a hip-opening stretch for the back leg.

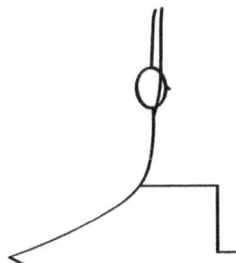

Warrior 2 - open your arms to the left and have them parallel to the floor reaching out with your fingers. Turn your back foot out slightly,

and make sure to align your front heel with the middle of the back foot. Bend your front leg at a 90-degree angle, and your back leg stays straight. Turn your head towards your front hand, and gaze over your middle finger.

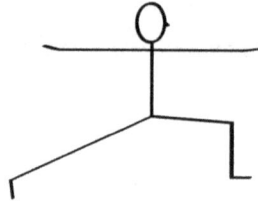

Reverse warrior - staying in Warrior 2 with the arms parallel with the floor; as you inhale, begin sliding your left hand along your back leg, while you reach up to the ceiling with your right arm. Eyes follow the rising hand. Make sure to keep your front leg bent at a 90-degree angle.

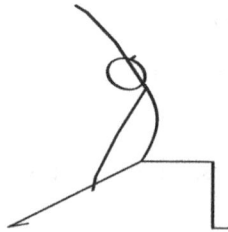

Side angle pose -take your right forearm and place it on your right thigh as you lift your left arm towards the ceiling. Try looking up at your left hand if you can. You should feel your entire left side body opening up.

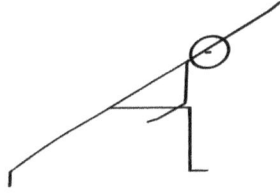

Runner's lunge – place hands down on either side of your right foot, right leg is at a 90-degree angle, while the left leg is extended and firm behind you, resting on the toes.

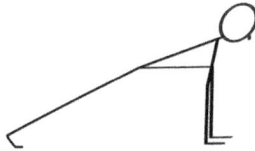

High plank - step the right leg back, hands under shoulders, feet hip-width apart, body parallel to the ground, core is tight, and shoulders are rolled back.

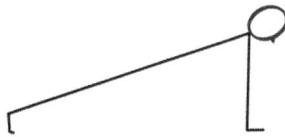

Lower yourself to the ground, leading with the chest and keeping your arms in, close to the body.

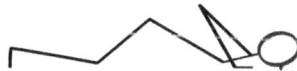

Upward dog - place hands at your sides at chest level with the lower body on the ground. Press into your hands and lift upper torso and hips off the ground; arms are straight, rolling the shoulders back and looking back for a slight backbend. Make sure the tops of the feet are touching the ground.

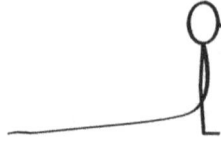

Downward dog – press back to the balls of your feet; hands on the ground shoulder-width apart; feet hip-width apart; the body is in a V; press the hips up and press the chest towards the thighs; your head should be between your arms.

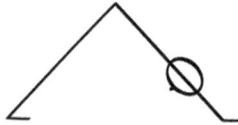

Forward hang – step feet forward to meet your hands, reaching your hands to the floor. Hang forward with a relaxed head.

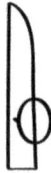

Mountain – inhale, as you stand tall with the arms overhead parallel to the ears, shoulders relaxed and away from the ears.

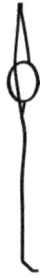

Repeat that sequence on the left side (Follow below)

Warrior 1 – step your left leg forward with the knee bent at a 90-degree angle, and the right leg is straight behind you with your right foot turned out slightly. Square your hips to face forward and reach your arms up parallel to your ears. This is a hip-opening stretch for the back leg.

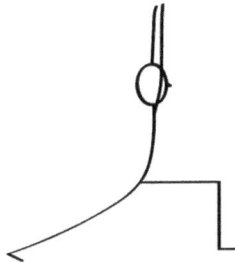

Warrior 2 - open your arms to the right and have them parallel to the floor reaching with your fingers. Turn your back foot out slightly, and make sure to align your front heel with the middle of your back foot. Bend your front leg at a 90-degree angle, and your back leg stays straight. Turn your head towards your front hand, and gaze over your middle finger.

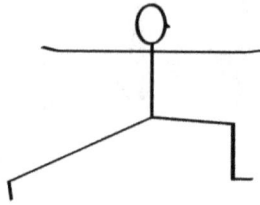

Reverse Warrior - staying in Warrior 2 with the arms parallel with the floor; as you inhale, begin sliding your right hand along your right leg while you reach up to the ceiling with your left arm. Eyes follow the rising hand. Make sure to keep your front leg bent at a 90-degree angle.

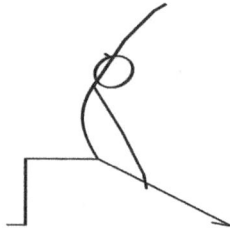

Side angle pose - take your left forearm and place it on your left thigh as you lift your right arm towards the ceiling. Try looking up at your right hand if you can. You should feel your entire right side opening up.

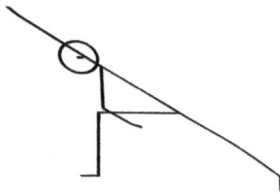

Runner's lunge – place your hands on the floor on either side of your left foot while your right leg is extended and firm behind you, with the toes on the ground.

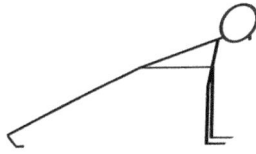

High plank – step your left leg back, hands under shoulders, feet hip-width apart, body is parallel to the ground, core is tight, and shoulders are rolled back.

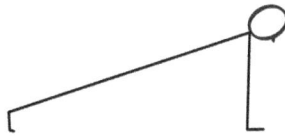

Lower yourself to the ground, leading with the chest and keeping your arms in, close to the body.

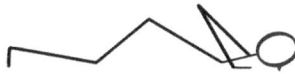

Upward dog - place hands at your sides at chest level with the lower body on the ground; press into your hands and lift upper torso and hips off the ground; arms are straight, rolling the shoulders back and looking back for a slight backbend. Make sure the tops of the feet are touching the ground.

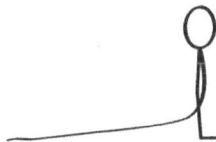

Downward dog – press back to the balls of your feet; hands on the ground shoulder-width apart; feet are hip-width apart; the body is in a

V; press the hips up and press the chest towards the thighs; your head should be between your arms.

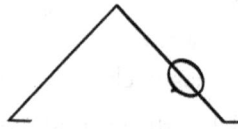

Forward hang – step your feet up to meet your hands, reaching your hands towards the ground. Hang forward with a relaxed head.

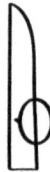

Mountain – inhale, as you stand tall with arms overhead parallel to the ears, and shoulders are relaxed.

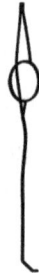

Sequence Four (Balance)

Warrior 3 – shift your weight to your right foot. Slowly bend forward as you bring your left leg up parallel with the floor; big toe facing the floor and press your heel away. Hands are at your sides as you look forward and balance on the right leg. You may have a slight bend in the knee to relieve tension.

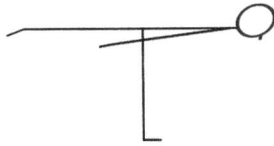

Standing leg split - place both hands on the ground and reach your left leg up as high as you can and hold.

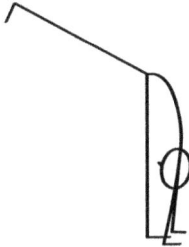

Half Moon - move your right hand one hand length to the right on the floor. Slowly turn your body to the left, as you begin to slowly lift your left arm off the ground. Begin reaching the arm straight up to the ceiling, as your leg is parallel with the floor, and the body is facing to the left. This is a challenging balance pose. See if you can hold for five seconds.

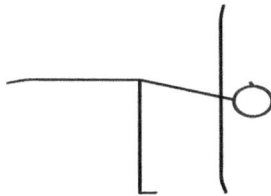

Repeat on the left side (See below)

Warrior 3 – shift your weight to your left foot. Slowly bend forward as you bring your right leg up parallel with the floor; big toe facing the floor and press your heel away. Hands are at your sides as you look forward and balance on the left leg. You may have a slight bend in the knee to relieve tension.

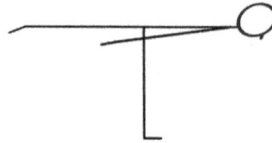

Standing leg split - place both hands on the ground and reach your right leg as high as you can. Hold for five seconds.

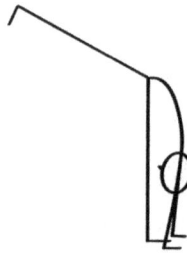

Half-moon - move your left hand one hand length to the left on the floor. Slowly turn your body to the right, as you begin to slowly lift your right arm off the ground. Begin reaching the arm straight up to the ceiling, as your leg is parallel to the floor, and your body is facing to the right. See if you can hold for five seconds.

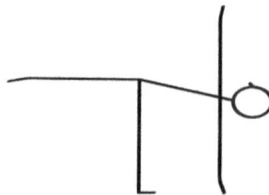

Tip of the day: Overcoming negative self-talk. To help overcome negative thinking, one strategy you could use is to immediately catch yourself and tell yourself: **"STOP IT"**. Then ask yourself this one simple question: "What would I say to my dear friend or to a person I care about deeply, if they said this to themselves"? After asking the question, see what answer comes to you, and imagine saying this to yourself! Sometimes it is easier if we look at something from someone else's perspective.

Focus of the day: If you don't accept or like yourself, it will be hard for anyone else to reciprocate that. What you put out there will be attracted to you. If you don't believe in yourself, you will not be successful! Accept yourself and be grateful for the life you have. Live in the moment and try not to let past mistakes eat away at you. When you speak negatively about yourself, ask yourself what your biggest fan would say to you instead.

Mindfulness Activity: Self -Critic and Self-Acceptance

In today's mindfulness exercise, we are going to listen to our inner critic. Let's take a moment to get into a comfortable position, and to allow ourselves to relax. Let's start out by taking three nice, big, deep breaths, in through our nose and out through our nose. Allow the body to settle in and to release all tension and tightness.

Now, I want you to think about the way you talk to yourself on a daily basis. What are the conversations that you are having with yourself? We will call this your inner critic. Our inner critic likes to speak negatively and harshly to us. We tend to have a lot of self-talk all the time. What I want you to know is that these critical thoughts we have are not necessarily truths.

So, take a moment to pick out the number one negative repeated thought that you have about yourself. Think of something you criticize yourself for. This could be something like, "I am not smart", "I am not good at anything", "No one likes me". These are examples of inner critic talk. Come up with your number one repetitive negative statement.

Now, ask this question, "Is this really true"? How could you look at this statement with some self-compassion? Is there any way you could turn this negative into a positive right now by being kind to yourself?

If you are having trouble with this, that is okay. If you cannot offer yourself some nice words, then think of what your loved one would say to you right now.

Take a moment to imagine cutting yourself some slack and being gentler with yourself, allowing for mistakes and recognizing that these mistakes only help us grow as humans.

I would like you to place both hands on your heart right now, and say these statements to yourself:

I am having a difficult time right now;

Everyone has difficult times.

May I be kind to myself at this moment.

May I give myself the compassion and understanding that I need.

I am worthy of love and acceptance.

I am worthy of happiness.

I want to be okay with myself and accept myself.

I know and realize that I must love myself first and treat myself with respect.

I will try to be kinder, nicer, and more forgiving of myself.

Take a moment to notice how you feel. When you are ready, take a long inhale, a long exhale, and open your eyes.

LESSON SEVEN

Yoga

※

Sequence One (Lay on Stomach)

Quad stretch - bend both knees, reach around to grab your feet or ankles, and press heels to your buttocks for a quad stretch. Hold for ten seconds.

Bow pose - reach for your ankles, flex your feet, and press your ankles into your hands as you lift your upper body and legs off the ground. Repeat two times and hold for ten seconds each.

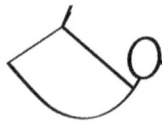

Superman - laying on your stomach with your arms at your sides and legs straight. Inhale, and as you exhale, lift your legs and arms up and hold for five seconds. Reach with the fingers and reach with the toes. Repeat five times.

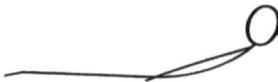

Windshield wipers- bend both knees and let your legs sway side to side to stretch the low back, keeping your torso and shoulders flat on the ground. Rest your chin on your hands.

Child's pose - sit with your buttocks on your heels and place your arms straight out in front of you, reaching on the floor, as your forehead touches the ground. Take three breaths here and relax.

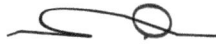

Sequence Two

Table-top – position yourself on the floor on your hands and knees, with your knees under your hips, and your hands under your shoulders.

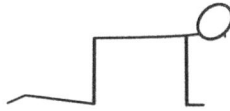

Cat cow – inhale, belly drops and chin lifts. Exhale, round the back and bring your chin to your chest. Repeat five times.

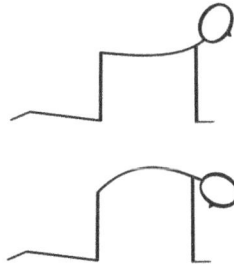

Dancing cat - begin to move your torso in slow circles in one direction, and then switch directions to open up and stretch the upper back. Make sure to keep your shoulders and hips still.

Downward dog – press back onto the balls of your feet; hands on the ground shoulder-width apart; feet are hip-width apart; the body is in a V; press the hips up and press the chest towards the thighs; your head should be between your arms.

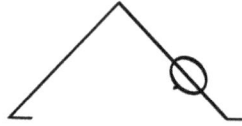

Walk the dog - pedal the heels, bending the right leg first and straightening the left, and then alternating to stretch the calves.

Forward hang – step feet up to meet hands, reaching your hands to the ground. Hang forward with a relaxed head.

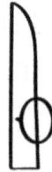

Mountain – inhale, as you stand tall with your arms overhead parallel to your ears, shoulders are relaxed and away from your ears.

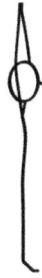

Sequence Three

Triangle pose right side- stand with legs four feet apart with right leg facing forward and left leg back with foot turned in to the right; legs are straight, and arms are parallel with the floor. Begin to hinge or bend from the waist forward over your right leg, and then windmill your arms so that your right hand is touching either your shin or the floor, and your left arm is reaching for the ceiling. Look up towards your hand if you can.

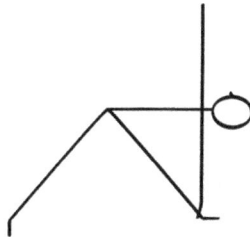

Reverse warrior - slowly come up and slide your left hand along your left leg as you reach your right arm up towards the ceiling and bend your right leg at a 90-degree angle.

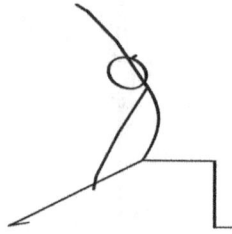

Moving between poses - move back and forth five times slowly between triangle pose and reverse warrior pose. Inhale to reverse warrior and exhale into triangle pose.

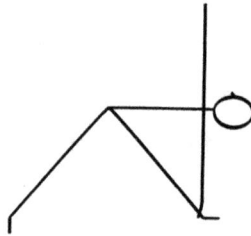

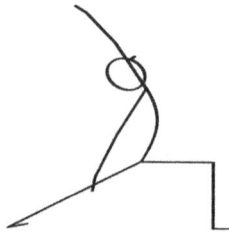

Mountain pose – stand with your feet hip-width apart and bring your arms parallel to your ears.

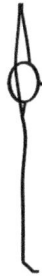

Pyramid pose – step your left leg back about one to two feet. With both legs straight, inhale and reach arms up, parallel to your ears, and as you exhale, reach forward over your right leg. Reach for your shin or the floor if you can, as you lean back for a hamstring stretch.

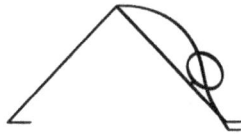

Wide-leg stretch - turn the body to the left with your hands on your hips. Stand with a wide stance and your toes pointing forward. Inhale and get taller, as you exhale, lean forward and reach for the floor. Walk hands to the right leg and hold; then walk hands to the left leg and hold.

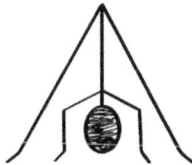

Forward hang – step feet together, reaching the hands towards the ground. Hang forward with a relaxed head.

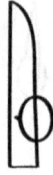

Rag doll - roll up like a rag doll to a standing position with the head being the last body part to lift.

Repeat on the other side (Follow below)

Triangle - stand with legs four feet apart with left leg facing forward and right leg back with foot turned in to the left; legs are straight, and arms are parallel with the floor. Begin to hinge or bend from the waist forward over your left leg and then windmill your arms so that your left hand is touching either your shin or the floor, and your right arm is reaching for the ceiling. See if you can look up at your hand.

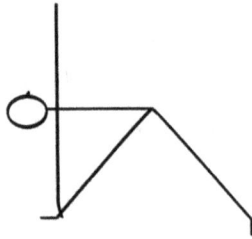

Reverse Warrior - slowly come up and slide your right hand along your right leg as you reach your left arm up and bend your left leg at a 90-degree angle. Eyes are looking at your left hand.

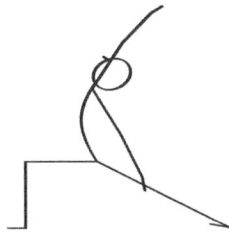

Moving between poses - move back and forth five times slowly between triangle pose and reverse warrior pose. Inhale to reverse warrior and exhale into triangle pose.

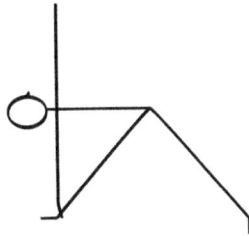

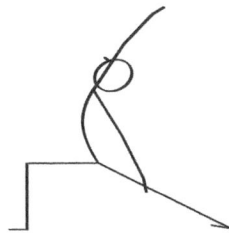

Mountain pose – stand with your feet hip-width apart and bring your arms parallel to your ears.

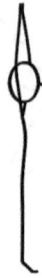

Pyramid pose – step your right leg back. With both legs straight, inhale and reach arms up, parallel to your ears, and as you exhale, reach forward over your left leg and reach for your shin or the floor if you can. Lean back for a hamstring stretch.

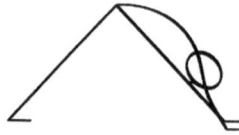

Wide- leg stretch - turn the body to the right with your hands on your hips. Stand with a wide stance and your toes pointing forward. Inhale and get taller, as you exhale, lean forward and reach for the floor. Walk hands to the right leg and hold; then walk hands to the left leg and hold.

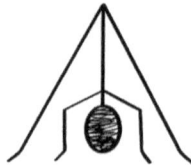

Forward hang – step feet together, reaching the hands towards the ground. Hang forward with a relaxed head.

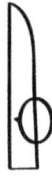

Rag doll – roll up like a rag doll to a standing position with the head being the last body part to lift.

Sequence Four

Mountain - stand tall with your feet hip-width apart, and your arms overhead parallel to your ears, shoulders are relaxed.

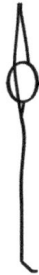

Forward hang - bend at the waist, reaching your hands towards the ground. Hang forward with a relaxed head.

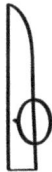

Half lift – inhale, as you slide hands along your shins with a straight back, upper torso coming up parallel to the ground.

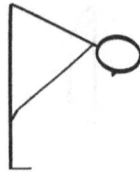

Forward hang – exhale, as you bend from the waist, reaching the hands towards the ground. Hang forward with a relaxed head.

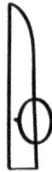

High plank – place hands on the ground under the shoulders, step legs back with toes on the ground, body is parallel to the floor, core is tight, and shoulders are rolled back.

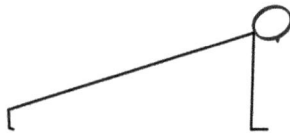

Lower yourself to the ground, leading with the chest and keeping your arms in, close to the body.

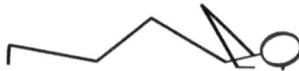

Upward dog - place hands at your sides at chest level with the lower body on the ground; press into your hands and lift upper torso and hips off the ground; arms are straight; rolling shoulders back and looking back for a slight backbend with the tops of the feet on the ground.

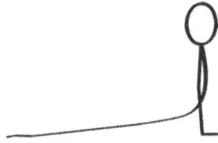

Downward dog – press back to the balls of your feet, with the feet hip-width apart; hands are shoulder width apart; the body is in a V; press the hips up and press the chest towards the thighs; your head should be between your arms.

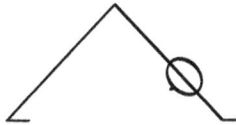

Child's pose - sit with your buttocks on your heels and place your arms straight out in front of you, reaching on the floor, as your forehead touches the ground.

Puppy pose – come into a table-top position, with your knees under your hips, and your hands under your shoulders. Start leaning your buttocks towards your heels and reach your arms forward on the ground. Make sure to keep your belly from resting on your thighs. You may rest your forehead on the ground if you can.

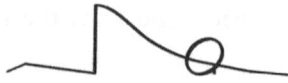

****Repeat sequence FOUR
one more time starting with mountain pose****

Sequence Five (Seated position with crossed legs or easy seat)

Chest and back stretch -interlace your fingers; palms are turned away from you, and as you inhale, extend your arms up to the ceiling. On your exhale, round your back, bringing your chin to your chest, lowering your arms to parallel with the ground, and press forward for an upper back stretch. Repeat this movement five times; inhaling as you reach up and exhaling as you press out.

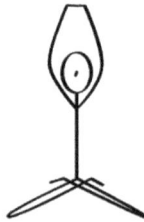

Seated side stretches - reach right arm up, and side bend over to the left. Then, reach left arm up, and side bend over to the right. Repeat three times on each side.

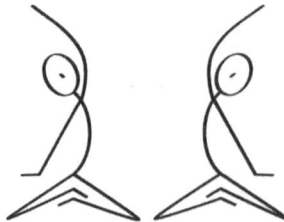

Seated pike position – legs are straight in front of you with feet together. Place your hands on the back of your head, and gently press your chin to your chest, and then return to starting position. Repeat this stretch five times.

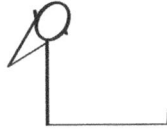

Butterfly position – place the soles of your feet together and reach forward with your arms.

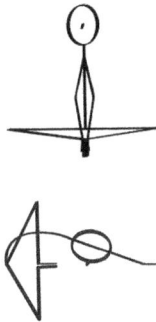

Tip of the day: Breathe and live in the moment. Start living your life from moment to moment. Don't get stuck in the past or be worried about the future, because all you have is right now. Use breathing as a tool to bring you back to reality.

Focus of the day: Learning about being mentally tough – To be mentally tough means you know how to deal with distractions. There are internal and external factors. External factors include friends, family, coaches, and teammates. Internal factors are your own thoughts and feelings about yourself. It is important to learn to focus on things you can control and stay in the moment! Take one moment at a time. One of the biggest challenges for most people (including athletes) is worrying about things that they cannot control. There are so many things that we cannot control. Our concentration should be on the things we can control, such as our ability to focus, our attitude, our effort level and our thoughts. It is important to realize that you cannot control other people's behavior. This means that you have no control over your opposing team, your coach, your fans, and the referees. Many athletes get angry, frustrated, and upset by the actions of others. This is out of your control! You can only control how you handle and respond to this! The most important part of a game is learning to focus, not allowing distractions to get in your way, and to continue to stay in the moment, giving your best effort.

Mindfulness Activity: Learning to Focus on One Thing at a Time (Mindful Schools, 2015)

Find a comfortable seated position. Close your eyes and take a moment to be still. Focus your attention on your breath, breathing naturally and normally in and out of your nose. Take a moment to allow yourself to relax, with nothing else to do.

Please bring your attention to your feet.

Can you try to feel your feet, and notice any sensations that may arise in your feet? When I talk about sensations, I am referring to such things as temperature (warmth or coolness), tingly sensations, heaviness or lightness, pulsing, itchiness, soreness and pain, or relaxation.

Now, bring your attention to one breath (an inhalation and exhaletion).

Now, bring your attention to your hands. Notice the feelings or sensations in your hands and how they feel.

Bring your attention to one breath (an inhalation and exhalation).

Now, bring your attention to your back. Notice how your back feels. From your lower back all the way up the spine to your upper back.

Bring your attention to one breath (an inhalation and exhalation).

Now, bring your attention to your stomach, and notice any sensations in your tummy.

Bring your attention to one breath (an inhalation and exhalation).

Now, bring your attention to your mind, and notice what thoughts are swirling around right now. Just notice.

Then, bring your attention back to one breath.

Next, bring your attention to sounds in the room right now. What sounds do you notice? Are they loud or subtle?

Then, bring your attention back to one breath.

Next, I want you to bring your attention to a wonderful, happy memory from your past. Take a moment to soak up the memory. It could be anything that makes you feel truly happy.

Now, bring your focus back to this room, listening to my voice.

Next, bring your focus to something you are looking forward to in the future. Take a moment to indulge in this excitement.

Now, bring your attention to one breath.

Next, bring your attention to your most memorable moment in your sport. Pick a time or play that stands out to you the most right now.

Then, bring your attention to one breath.

Lastly, bring to your mind an image of yourself performing at your very best. See yourself and visualize it clearly in your mind. What is it that you want to accomplish? Hold on to that image for a moment and notice how it feels when you visualize yourself performing at your best.

Bring your attention to one breath.

And when you are ready, you can open your eyes.

LESSON EIGHT

Yoga

Sequence One (Seated position)

Twist right – inhale, as you bring both arms up parallel to the ears and exhale, twisting body to the right with right arm behind you and left arm in front of you, resting on the floor.

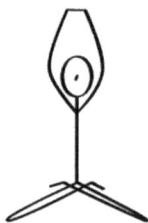

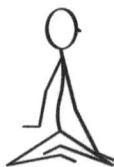

Twist left – inhale, both arms up parallel to the ears and exhale, twisting body to the left with the left arm behind you and the right arm in front of you, resting on the floor.

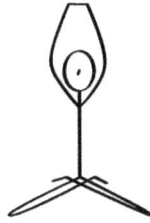

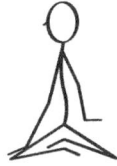

Repeat the twists two more times.

Side bend right - bring the left arm up, parallel to your ear, and then exhale as you bring the arm over to the right, opening the left-side body.

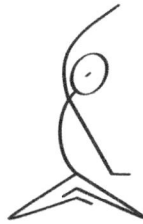

Side bend left - bring the right arm up, parallel to your ear, and then exhale as you bring the arm over to the left, opening the right-side body.

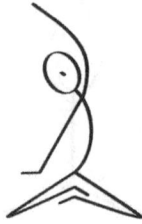

Repeat two more times.

Neck stretch right - bring right ear to the right shoulder and hold for five seconds.

Neck stretch left - bring left ear to left shoulder and hold for five seconds.

Repeat two more times on each side.

Butterfly stretch – place the soles of the feet together, and lean forward, reaching out with your arms and hands. Try to press your knees towards the floor.

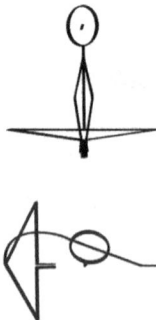

Reverse table-top – get into a seated position. Place your feet on the ground hip-width apart, and bring your hands behind you, resting flat on the ground shoulder-width apart; fingertips should face your feet.

Press your feet into the floor, lift your hips, and roll your shoulders and chest open, bringing your head back. Hold for at least 5 seconds. Repeat this pose two more times.

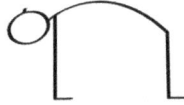

Child's pose - sit with your buttocks on your heels, reaching your arms forward, placing your forehead on the ground.

Cow pose – get into table-top position on all fours, inhale as you drop your belly, roll your shoulders back, open your chest, and lift your chin.

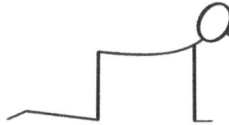

Downward dog – press back onto the balls of your feet; hands on the ground shoulder-width apart, feet are hip-width apart; the body is in a V; press the hips up and press the chest towards the thighs; your head should be between your arms.

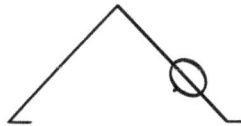

Forward fold – step the feet forward to meet the hands, reaching the arms and hands towards the ground. Hang forward with a relaxed head.

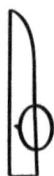

Half lift – inhale, as you slide your hands along your shins with a straight back, upper torso coming up parallel to the ground.

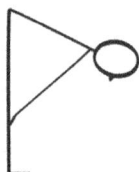

Forward fold – exhale, and bend at the waist, reaching hands towards the floor, and hang forward with a relaxed head.

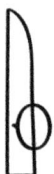

High Plank – place your hands on the ground shoulder-width apart, step your feet back hip-width apart, resting on the toes; core is tight, and shoulders are rolled back.

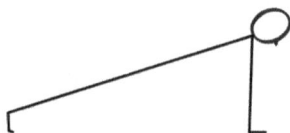

Lower yourself to the ground, leading with the chest and keeping your arms in, close to the body.

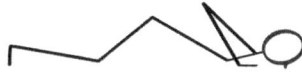

Upward dog - place hands at your sides at chest level with the lower body on the ground; press into your hands and lift upper torso and hips off the ground; arms are straight, rolling the shoulders back and looking back for a slight backbend with the tops of the feet resting on the floor.

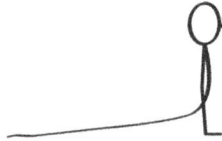

Downward dog – press back onto the balls of your feet; hands are on the ground shoulder-width apart; feet are hip-width apart; the body is in a V; press the hips up and press the chest towards the thighs; your head should be between your arms.

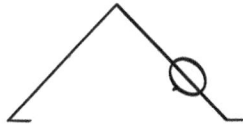

Repeat sequence one more time starting with cow pose into a downward dog.

Sequence Two

Chair pose – stand with your knees and feet together, bend the knees and pretend you are sitting back in an imaginary chair. Weight should be in your heels, and you are squeezing your inner thighs together. Bring your arms up, parallel to your ears. Focus on the strength in your lower body.

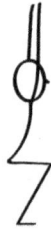

Twisting Chair right - press your inner thighs together, bring hands to your heart with the palms touching, and twist the body to the right as you bring your left elbow on the outside of your right upper leg. Press into the outer thigh for an extra twist to the right. Come back to chair pose.

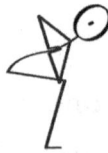

Twisting Chair left - press your inner thighs together, bring your hands to your heart with your palms touching, and twist body to the left as you bring your right elbow on the outside of your left upper leg. Press into the leg for an extra twist to the left.

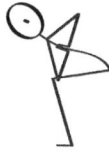

Forward fold - bend at the waist, reaching your hands towards the ground. Hang forward with a relaxed head.

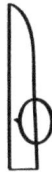

Runners lunge – place your hands on the ground, step your right leg back to a runners lunge. Left leg is bent at a 90-degree angle with the knee and ankle aligned, right leg is as extended and straight behind you as you can, resting on the toes. Hands are on either side of your left foot. Hold for three breaths.

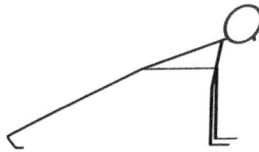

Low lunge – rest the right leg on the ground with knee and the top of the foot resting on the floor. Press the hip into the floor. Hold for three breaths.

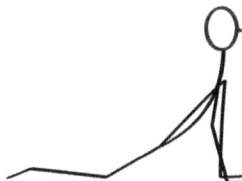

Runners lunge - bring the right leg back up off the ground and onto the toes. Hold for three breaths.

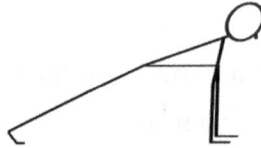

Crescent lunge - keep legs in runners lunge as you lift hands off the ground and bring the arms up so that they are parallel to your ears. Lift your right heel off the ground and keep your front leg bent at a 90-degree angle. Hold for three breaths.

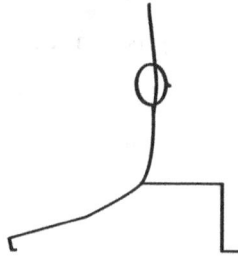

Forward fold – step foot forward, bend at the waist, reaching your hands towards the ground. Hang forward with a relaxed head.

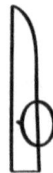

Rag doll – roll up like a rag doll to standing position, head being the last to lift.

Repeat on the other side (follow below)

Chair pose – stand with your knees and feet together, bend the knees and pretend you are sitting back in an imaginary chair. Weight should be in your heels and bring your arms up, parallel to your ears. Squeeze your inner thighs together and focus on the strength in your lower body.

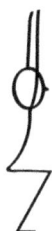

Twisting Chair right - press your inner thighs together, bring your hands to your heart with the palms touching, and twist body to the right as you bring your left elbow on the outside of your right upper leg. Press into the leg for an extra twist to the right. Come back to chair pose.

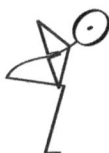

Twisting Chair left - press your inner thighs together, bring your hands to your heart and twist body to the left as you bring your right elbow on the outside of your left upper leg. Press into the leg for an extra twist to the left.

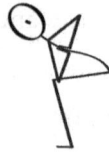

Forward fold - bend at the waist and hang forward with a relaxed head.

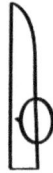

Runners lunge – bring your hands to the ground and step your left leg back to a runners lunge. Your right leg is bent at a 90-degree angle with the knee and ankle aligned. Left leg is as extended and straight behind you as you can with the toes on the ground. Hands are at either side of your right foot. Hold for three breaths.

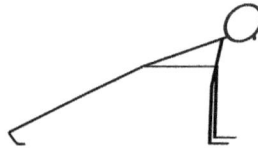

Low lunge - rest the left leg on the ground with the knee and the top of the foot resting on the floor. Press the hip into the floor. Hold for three breaths.

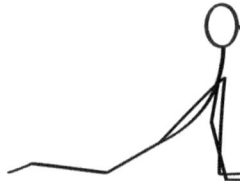

Runners lunge - bring the left leg back up off the ground and onto the toes. Hold for three breaths.

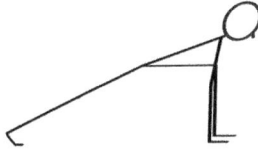

Crescent lunge - keep legs in runners lunge as you lift hands off the ground and bring the arms up parallel to your ears. Lift your left heel off the ground and keep your front leg bent at a 90-degee angle. Hold for three breaths.

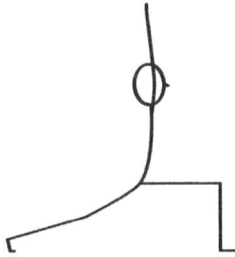

Forward fold – step leg forward, bend at the waist, and hang forward with a relaxed head.

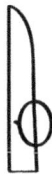

Rag doll – roll up like a rag doll to a standing position, the head being the last to lift.

Sequence Three

Table-top – get on the floor on your hands and knees, with your knees under your hips, and your hands under your shoulders.

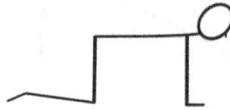

Cat cow – inhale, belly drops and chin lifts. Exhale, round the back and bring your chin to your chest. Repeat five times.

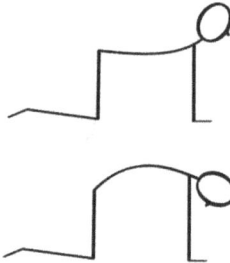

Child's pose – sit back with your buttocks on your heels and reaching arms forward, placing your forehead on the ground.

Puppy pose – come into a table-top position with the knees under hips, and hands under shoulders. Start leaning your buttocks towards your heels and reach your arms forward on the ground for a spine and shoulder stretch. Make sure your belly does not rest on your thighs. You may rest your forehead on the ground.

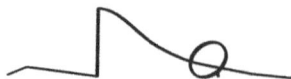

Tip of the day: Self-Care - You need to take care of yourself, both mentally and physically. Examples include; eating well, not over-training, stretching, hydrating, getting enough sleep, being kind to yourself, and surrounding yourself with positive people.

Focus of the day: Focus on you! You are important, and to be your best self, you need to take extra care of your physical and mental well-being. Make sure to be strong in all five components of fitness (muscular strength, muscular endurance, cardiovascular endurance, flexibility, and body composition). Also, make sure to surround yourself with people in your life who make you feel valued and worthy. Negativity breeds negativity, and the same goes for positivity. If you are always around people who complain, are negative, always look at the worst-case scenario, you most likely will begin to feel the same way. If there is a chance to let go of some of those people in your life, it would be beneficial to your mental health to do so.

Mindfulness Activity: Love and Kindness for Yourself and a Loved One

Please find a comfortable seat in a mindful body position, sitting comfortably with the spine long and straight, shoulders relaxed, and hands resting in your lap. Now, take a deep breath in through the nose and out through the nose. Allow your body to let go, relax, unwind, and be at peace. We are going to offer ourselves some kind words and phrases, and then we will offer those kind words and phrases to others we care about. First, I want you to imagine sitting near a beautiful lake. Imagine you are seated on a cozy bench right near the edge of this beautiful lake. Take a moment to enjoy this scenery. Now, I want you to lean forward, and see your reflection in this lake. Your reflection is crystal clear. As you are looking at your reflection, I want you to say the following phrases to yourself:

May I be happy

May I be filled with joy in my life

May I be healthy in my mind and my body

May I be safe and feel secure

May I have the strength to handle difficult situations

Take a moment to sit back on your bench and take in the beautiful lake view again. Take a deep breath in and a deep breath out. Now, I want you to bring to mind someone who you care about deeply. I want you to imagine this person doing something that they love to do. Picture this person feeling happy, smiling, and having a great time. You start to feel happy and peaceful, seeing how your loved one is enjoying him/herself. Now, I want you to imagine that this person who you care about joins you on your bench near the lake. Imagine that your loved one sits down next to you, and you turn to face him/her. Please imagine repeating these statements to this person:

May you be happy

May you be filled with joy in your life

May you be healthy in your mind and your body

May you be safe and feel secure

May you have the strength to handle difficult situations

After saying these statements to your loved one, he/she begins to smile, and look at you with such love and appreciation. You can feel the love between the two of you, and it brings a smile to your face as well.

Now, imagine that the two of you turn to face the lake again, soaking up the beauty this lake has to offer. You sit in stillness and silence with the one you love, feeling compassion, kindness, hope, and gratitude for being you, and for having the love and support from this person.

Take a moment to bring your attention back to your breathing. Taking a nice big inhalation, and a big exhalation. When you are ready, you can open your eyes.

LESSON NINE

Yoga

Sequence One

Wide child's pose - separate knees wider than hips as you sit your buttocks on your heels and extend your arms and hands to reach forward on the floor.

Cat cow – come into a table-top position with your knees under your hips and your hands under your shoulders. Inhale, as your belly drops and chin lifts. Exhale, as you round the back and bring your chin to your chest. Repeat five times.

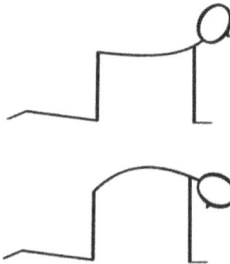

Downward dog – hands on the ground shoulder-width apart, lift your knees off the ground and step the feet back so that they are hip-width apart; the body is in a V; press your hips up and press your chest towards your thighs; your head should be between your arms.

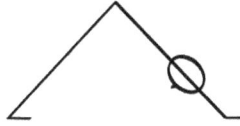

Walk the dog - pedal the heels right and left to stretch the calves.

Forward hang – step feet forward, bend at the waist, reaching your hands towards the floor. Hang forward with a relaxed head.

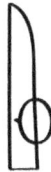

Wide leg forward bend - separate your feet as far as you can with toes pointed straight. Hands are reaching for the floor in the center.

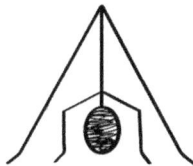

Twist right - place your left hand on the ground directly under your face as you lift the right arm up to the ceiling and only twist your upper torso. Try not to sway your hips in this position. Return to center.

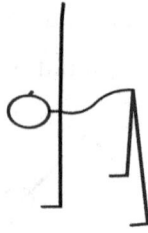

Twist left - place your right hand on the ground directly under your face as you lift the left arm up to the ceiling and only twist your upper torso without shifting your weight or moving your hips. Come back to center.

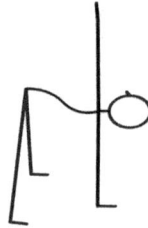

Wide leg with chest expansion - interlace fingers and raise your arms behind you, reaching the arms up as high as you can for a chest expansion.

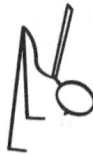

Downward dog – place your hands on the ground shoulder-width apart; step feet back hip-width apart; the body is in a V; press the hips up and press the chest towards the thighs; your head should be between your arms.

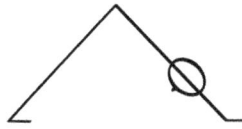

Right runners lunge - step right leg forward in a lunge position at a 90-degree angle. Hands are on either side of your right foot, with the knee over the ankle. The back leg is extended and firm, resting on the toes.

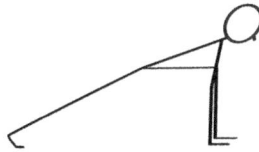

Low runners lunge - lower the left leg to the ground, resting the knee and top of the foot on the floor for a hip stretch.

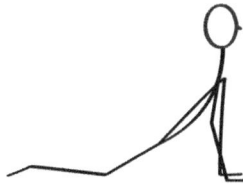

Lizards pose (lunge with a forearm stretch) - bring your hands to the inside of the right foot and lower your forearms to the ground if you can. Let your right leg fan-out. Hold for five seconds. Return hands to either side of your right foot.

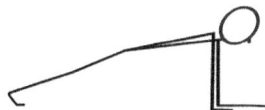

Calf and shin stretch - shift hips back and straighten the right leg as you reach your buttocks towards your left heel, but do not sit on your heel. Point and flex your right foot for a shin and calf stretch.

One-leg hamstring stretch – now, sit with your buttocks on your left heel and keep right leg extended long in front of you on the ground with your toes pointed up. Inhale, and reach your arms up to the ceiling. As you exhale, lean forward over your right leg, reaching your hands towards your foot for a one-leg hamstring stretch.

Downward dog – place your hands on the ground shoulder-width apart; step feet back hip-width apart; the body is in a V; press the hips up and press the chest towards the thighs; your head should be between your arms.

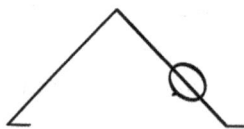

Left runners lunge - step left leg forward in a lunge position at a 90-degree angle. Hands are on either side of your left foot, with the knee over the ankle. The back leg is extended and firm, resting on the toes.

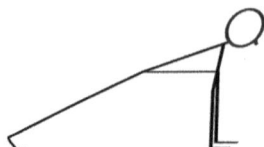

Low runners lunge - lower the right leg to the ground, with the knee and top of the foot resting on the floor. Sink into the hips.

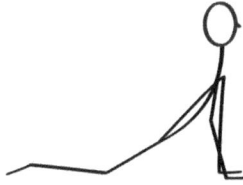

Lizards pose (lunge with a forearm stretch)- bring your hands to the inside of left foot and lower your forearms to the ground, if you can. Let your left leg fan-out. Hold for five seconds. Return hands to either side of your left foot.

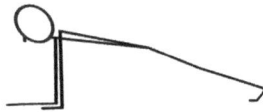

Calf and shin stretch - shift hips back and straighten the left leg as you reach your buttocks towards your right heel, but do not rest on your heel. Point and flex foot your left foot for a shin and calf stretch.

One-leg hamstring stretch – now, sit with your buttocks on your right heel and keep left leg extended long in front of you on the ground with the toes pointed up. Inhale, and reach your arms up to the ceiling. As you exhale, lean forward over your left leg, reaching your hands towards your foot for a one-leg hamstring stretch.

Downward dog – hands on the ground shoulder-width apart; step feet back hip-width apart; the body is in a V; press the hips up and press the chest towards the thighs; your head should be between your arms.

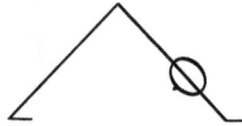

Forward fold – step feet up, bend at the waist, and hang forward with a relaxed head.

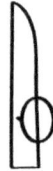

Sequence Two (Seated Position)

Single cow pose - cross right leg over left leg so that your knees are lined up, and your feet are near your buttocks- grab the tops of your feet and then give your arches of your feet a foot rub.

Lean forward for a glute, and hip stretch, reaching your arms and hands out as far as you can. Hold for ten seconds.

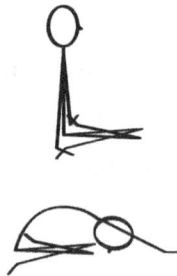

Single cow pose - cross left leg over right leg so that your knees are lined up, bring your feet towards buttocks, and place your fingers between your toes and massage your toes. Lean forward for a glute, and hip stretch, reaching your arms and hands as far as you can. Hold for ten seconds.

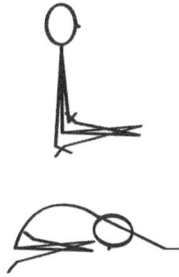

Pike stretch – place your legs out in front of you extended long. Inhale, as you reach your arms towards the ceiling, and exhale, as you reach your hands towards your feet. Repeat these five times, inhaling as you reach up, and exhaling as you reach forward.

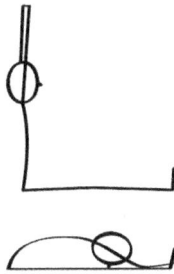

Straddle stretch – separate and widen your legs as far as you can comfortably go. Inhale, reaching your arms up to the ceiling, and exhale, reaching your hands on the floor in front of you for an inner thigh stretch. Repeat these five times, inhaling as you reach up, and exhaling as you reach forward.

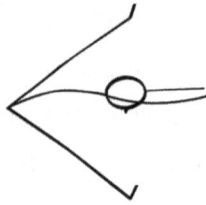

Tip of the day: Be grateful for all that you have in life!

Focus of the day: Gratitude is such an important part of our lives. Being, and feeling grateful allows us to appreciate everything that has been given to us and can make us feel happier.

Mindfulness Activity: Feeling Gratitude

Let's take a moment to settle into our mindful body position, seated upright, comfortable, spine elongated, shoulders down, body soft and relaxed. Take a breath in and try to extend your exhale. Let's try this again. Take a deep breath in, and then slowly exhale the air out. One more time, take a deep breath in through the nose and slowly exhale through your nose. Try to let go of everything right now. There is nothing you need to do, nowhere you need to be, because everything you need is right here at this moment with me.

Let's shift our attention to gratitude. Take a moment to be grateful that you woke up today and have this day. Let's say to ourselves, "I am grateful for this day."

Let's be grateful that we have our bodies that allow us to do all sorts of things like walking, running, biking, and playing sports. Let's say to ourselves, "I am grateful for my body."

Let's take a moment to be grateful for our minds. We are able to think, create, imagine, visualize, and study with our minds. Let's say to ourselves, "I am grateful for my mind."

Now, let's take a moment to be grateful for our health. If you don't have your health, then nothing else matters. Let's say to ourselves, "I am grateful for my health."

Let's take a moment to be grateful for those around you who love you. Be grateful that you are loved and have people in your life who care about you. Take a moment to think of one or two people in your life who care about you deeply. Be grateful you have that love. Notice how it feels in your body when you think of this person who loves you.

Let's take a moment to be grateful for your home, the roof over your head that provides shelter. Let's say to ourselves, "I am grateful for my home."

Let's take a moment to be grateful for all the opportunities that you have in your life. You have the choice to pursue any opportunity that comes your way. Be grateful for having choices in your life. Let's say to ourselves, "I am grateful for choices."

Let's be grateful for our team and the comradery that this team represents.

Let's be grateful for our lives, just the way they are. We have so much to be grateful for and appreciate in life.

Now, take a moment to notice how you feel. Perhaps you are feeling thankful and appreciative.

Take a deep breath, in through your nose and a deep breath out through your nose, and slowly open your eyes.

LESSON TEN

Yoga

Sequence One

Mountain -stand tall with the feet hip-width apart, and your arms overhead parallel to your ears. Shoulders are relaxed and away from the ears.

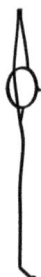

Forward fold - bend at the waist, reaching your hands towards the ground. Hang forward with a relaxed head.

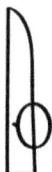

Half lift – inhale, as you slide your hands along the shins with a straight back, upper torso coming up parallel to the ground.

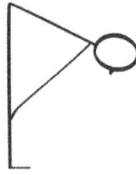

Forward fold – exhale, as you bend at the waist and hang forward with a relaxed head.

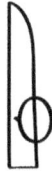

Downward dog – place your hands on the ground shoulder-width apart; step feet back hip-width apart; the body is in a V; press the hips up and press the chest towards the thighs; your head should be between your arms.

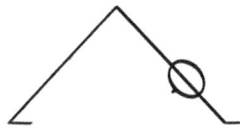

Walk the dog - pedal the heels right and left to stretch the calves.

Three leg dog - lift your right leg up as high as you can.

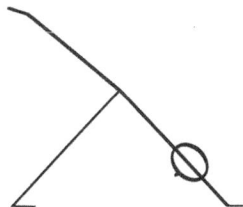

Runners Lunge - swing the leg forward to a right runners lunge, with the right leg at a 90-degree angle. Knee and ankle are aligned. Hands are on either side of your foot. Back leg is extended and firm with the toes on the ground.

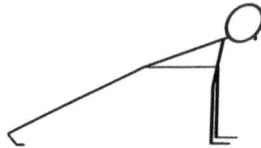

Warrior 2 – stand up and open your upper body to the left; arms are parallel to the floor reaching with the fingers; right arm is facing forward and left arm is back. Turn your back foot out slightly, and make sure your front heel is in line with the middle of your back foot. Bend your front leg at a 90-degree angle. Your back leg stays straight. Turn your head to gaze over your front middle finger.

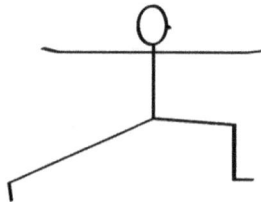

Reverse warrior - lean back and slide your left hand along the left leg, as your right arm reaches for the ceiling. Eyes follow the rising arm. Keep your front leg bent at a 90-degree angle.

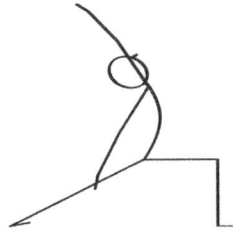

Side angle pose – move forward and place your right forearm on your right thigh. Extend your left arm up towards the ceiling and look up at your hand.

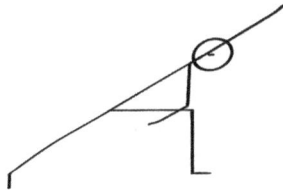

Triangle pose – lift your torso up, straighten both legs, and arms come up parallel to the floor. Hinge, or lean forward with your upper body from the waist over your right leg. Windmill your arms so that your right hand is reaching towards your shin or the floor, and the left arm reaches up.

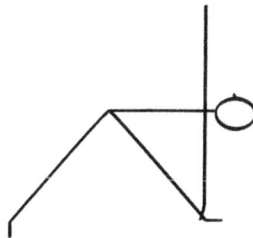

Wide leg forward fold – turn your body to face forward with toes pointing straight. Walk your feet wide, and bend from the waist, reaching your hands to the ground. Feel the stretch through the back of your legs.

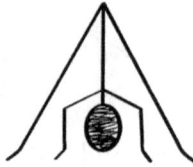

Shifting weight - move back and forth shifting your weight from your heels to your toes. Repeat the shifting back and forth six times.

Right runners lunge – turn your body to the right, bring your hands back to the ground on either side of your right foot. Bend your right leg at a 90-degree angle and extend your left leg straight behind you with your toes on the ground.

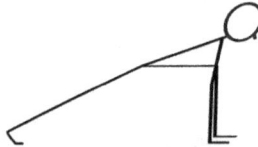

High Plank – step right leg back, hands under shoulders, feet hip-width apart, core is tight, and shoulders are rolled back.

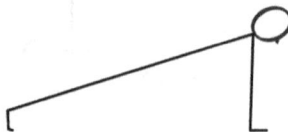

Lower yourself to the ground, leading with the chest and keeping your arms in, close to the body.

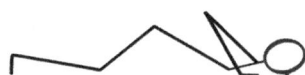

Upward dog - place hands at your sides at chest level with the lower body on the ground; press into your hands and lift upper torso and hips off the ground; arms are straight, roll the shoulders back and look back for a slight backbend, with the tops of the feet resting on the floor.

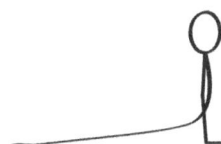

Downward dog – press back to the balls of your feet; hands on the ground shoulder-width apart; feet hip-width apart; the body is in a V; press the hips up and press the chest towards the thighs; your head should be between your arms.

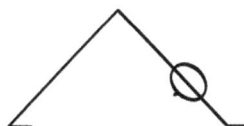

Repeat sequence on the other leg (follow below)

Three leg dog - lift your left leg up as high as you can.

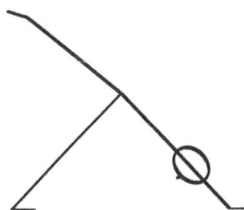

Runners lunge - swing your leg forward to a left runners lunge. Left leg is bent at a 90-degree angle with the knee over the ankle. Hands are on either side of your left foot, and your right leg is extended and straight behind you with the toes on the ground.

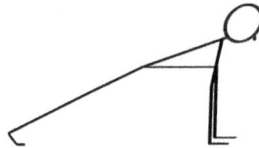

Warrior 2 - stand up and open your upper body to the right. Arms are parallel to the floor reaching with the fingers. Turn your back foot out slightly, and make sure to align your front heel with the middle of your back foot. Bend your front leg at a 90-degree angle, and your back leg stays straight.

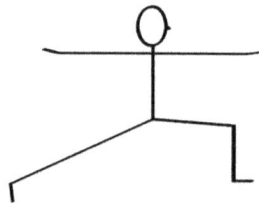

Reverse warrior - lean back and slide your right hand along your right leg. Your left arm reaches for the ceiling as your eyes follow the hand. Make sure to bend the left leg at a 90-degree angle.

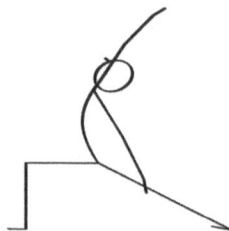

Side angle pose – move forward and place your left forearm on your left thigh, as you extend the right arm up and try looking at your right hand.

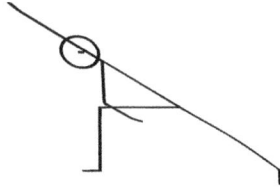

Triangle pose – lift your torso up and straighten both legs. Arms come up parallel to the floor. Hinge, or lean forward with your upper body from the waist over your left leg. Windmill the arms so that your left hand reaches for your shin or the floor, and your right arm reaches up towards the ceiling; eyes follow the rising hand.

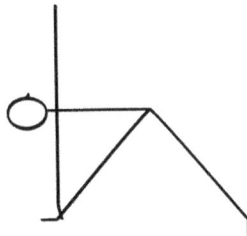

Wide leg forward fold - turn your body to face forward with the toes pointing forward. Walk your feet wide and reach your hands to the ground. Feel the stretch through the back of your legs.

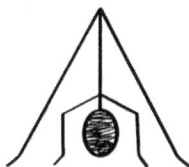

Shifting weight – move back and forth shifting your weight from your heels to your toes. Repeat this shifting back and forth six times.

Left runners lunge – turn your body to the left and bring your hands to the ground on either side of your left foot. Your left leg is bent at a 90-degree angle. Your right leg is extended and firm behind you with the toes on the ground.

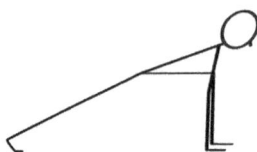

High Plank – step the left leg back; hands under shoulders; feet hip-width apart; core is tight; and shoulders are rolled back.

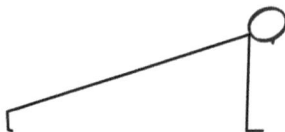

Lower yourself to the ground, leading with the chest and keeping your arms in, close to the body.

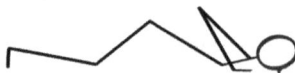

Upward dog - place hands at your sides at chest level with the lower body on the ground; press into your hands and lift upper torso and hips off the ground; arms are straight; roll the shoulders back and look back for a slight backbend, with the tops of the feet on the ground.

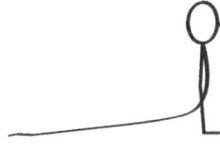

Downward dog – press back to the balls of your feet; hands on the ground shoulder-width apart; feet are hip-width apart; the body is in a V; press the hips up and press the chest towards the thighs; your head should be between your arms.

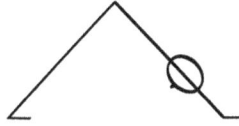

Child's pose – sit back with your buttocks on your heels, reaching your arms and hands forward. You can place your forehead on the ground if you can.

Sequence Two (Seated Position)

Reclined pigeon (figure four) - place the right ankle on left knee and sit up tall. Left foot is on the ground, try to bring the foot closer to your buttocks, and your hands are on the ground behind you under your shoulders. Roll the shoulders back, open the chest, and hold for three breaths.

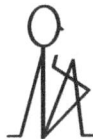

One-leg hamstring stretch - straighten the left leg on the ground and keep the right ankle on the left knee. Lean forward, reaching your hands towards your foot for a seated hamstring stretch.

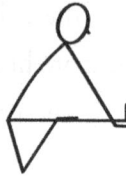

Seated twist - bend the right leg bringing the right knee to the chest and twist the body to the right for a spinal twist.

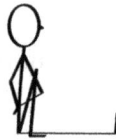

Reclined pigeon (figure four) – place the left ankle on the right knee and sit up tall. The right foot is on the ground, try to get the foot as close to the buttocks as you can. Hands are on the ground behind you under your shoulders. Roll the shoulders back, open the chest, and hold for three breaths.

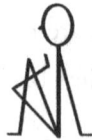

One-leg hamstring stretch - straighten the right leg on the ground and keep the left ankle on the right knee. Lean forward, reaching your hands towards your foot for seated hamstring stretch.

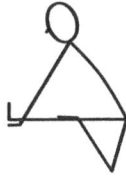

Seated twist - bend the left leg bringing the left knee into the chest and twist the body to the left for a spinal twist.

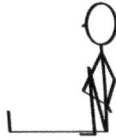

Sequence Three (Laying on back)

Low back stretch – bring the knees into the chest and rock side to side.

One-leg low back stretch - bring the right knee in to the chest and keep the left leg long on the ground.

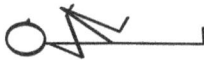

Spinal twist - bring the right arm out on the floor like a T, take the left hand and grab the right knee as you twist the right leg across your body to the left side for a twist.

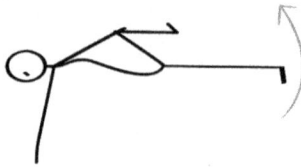

Low back stretch - bring both knees into the chest and rock side to side.

One-leg low back stretch - bring the left knee in to the chest and keep the right leg long on the ground.

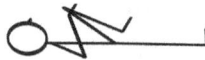

Spinal twist - bring the left arm out on the floor like a T, take the right hand and grab the left knee as you twist the left leg across your body to the right side.

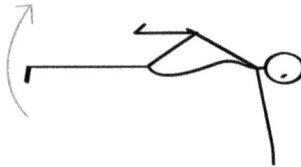

Double hamstring stretch - bring both legs straight up towards the ceiling, lift the head, neck and shoulders off the ground, and try to grab behind knees for a hamstring stretch. Repeat three times.

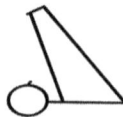

Tip of the day: Stop Worrying! There is no good that comes out of worrying, and it only hurts you.

Focus of the day: What is worry? Worrying is an anxious word, and it means to be concerned or nervous about something. Most of what we worry about doesn't happen anyway. The more we worry, the more anxious we become, and we begin to obsess about all different types of made-up scenarios in our minds. Worry only causes more stress and can lead to physical illness if we continue to get caught up in our worries. Worrying fuels stress and negative thinking. We usually have a narrative in our head about all the possible bad things that may happen to us. Worrying causes physical changes in the body, such as increased heart rate, increased blood pressure, and more rapid breathing. All of these physical symptoms put a strain on our bodies.

Mindfulness Activity: Finding Your Peaceful Place

Find a comfortable position where you can be still. Allow your body to relax and settle into your position. Let's begin by taking three slow, deep breaths, allowing our bodies to begin to relax. With each breath you take, try to visualize breathing in peace and calm, and breathing out tension and worry. Continue to breathe like this for three more breaths, breathing in peace and calm, and breathing out tension and worry.

As you settle into your body and your breath, let's begin you to create a picture in your mind of a beautiful, magical, peaceful place. This place could be anywhere in the world. It is a place that you are creating in your mind right now that makes you feel safe, secure, happy, and peaceful. Take a moment to look all around you, inviting in all of the details of this wonderful place you have created.

Let's start out by imagining what you can see. Look around and notice what your eyes can see. Perhaps there are trees, water, flowers, animals, or other people. See if you can notice the colors in this place, the amount of light or darkness in this place, the objects and landscapes that make up your magical place. Take it all in, enjoying the beauty of your peaceful place.

Now, let's notice any sounds in your peaceful place. What do you hear? Are the sounds loud or barely noticeable? Can you notice any smells or aromas in your peaceful place? Perhaps the smell of the ocean or fresh flowers, or perhaps the smell of a certain type of food? Just try to imagine what scents you are detecting in this place.

Now, see if you can imagine how you feel when you are visualizing this peaceful place. Do you feel relaxed, calm, happy, blissful, grateful, hopeful? Take a moment to allow those feelings to grow inside you. This magical place is taking you away from all your stress, worries, and responsibilities in life. This is a place where you feel free, alive, and happy. Imagine this peaceful place is the sanctuary that you can visit anytime you want, when you feel you need a break. This place is beautiful, calming, relaxing, peaceful, and tranquil. You are enjoying every moment you are spending in this place.

This magical place makes you feel on top of the world and untouchable. You feel proud, confident, happy, motivated, excited, and grateful. Take a moment to allow those feelings to grow and spread in your mind and in your body.

Then, take one more moment to look around you in this place, soaking up every last second of perfection in this peaceful place. (Pause)

Bring your attention now to your breathing, following each inhalation and exhalation. Bring your attention to how your body feels, and when you are ready, please open your eyes.

LESSON ELEVEN

Yoga

✴

Sequence One

Child's pose – sit back with your buttocks on your heels and reach your arms and hands forward.

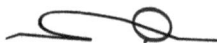

Cat cow – come into a table-top position with your knees under your hips, and your hands under your shoulders. Inhale, as you drop the belly and lift the chin. Exhale, as you round the back and bring your chin to your chest. Repeat five times.

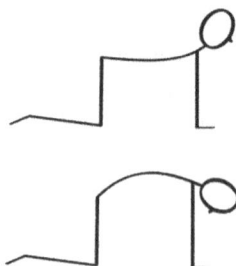

Downward dog – lift the knees up; press back onto the balls of your feet; hands on ground shoulder-width apart; feet are hip-width apart; the body is in a V; press the hips up and press the chest towards the thighs; your head should be between your arms.

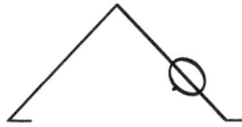

Forward fold – step feet forward, bend at the waist, reaching the hands towards the ground. Hang forward with a relaxed head.

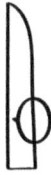

Half lift – inhale, as you slide your hands along your shins with a straight back. Upper torso comes up parallel to the ground.

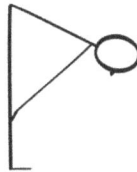

Crouching fold – exhale, as you bend down reaching your hands towards the ground; come into a tuck position and bring your chin to your chest.

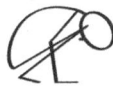

Half lift – extend the legs, as you slide your hands along your shins with a straight back; upper torso is parallel to the ground.

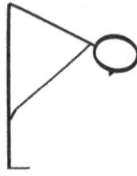

Forward fold - bend at the waist, reaching the hands towards the ground. Hang forward with a relaxed head.

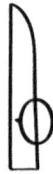

Mountain - stand tall with the arms overhead parallel to your ears, and shoulders are relaxed.

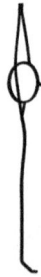

Half-moon to right - stand with knees and feet together; squeeze your inner thighs; bring your arms up so that they are parallel to your ears and interlace your fingers. Inhale, reach up, and get taller. Exhale, and lean to the right as you squeeze your inner thighs together and open your chest. Return to center position.

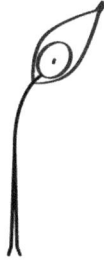

Half-moon to left - stand with the knees and feet together; squeeze your inner thighs together. Inhale, reach up, and get taller. Exhale, and lean to the left as you squeeze your inner thighs together and open your chest. Return to center position.

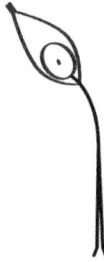

Baby back bend - lean back slightly with arms up, pressing hips forward for a slight back bend.

Hands at heart - palms together at chest level.

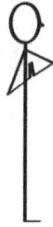

Forward fold – bend at the waist, reaching your hands towards the ground. Gently shake your head yes and shake your head no to release the neck.

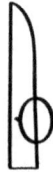

Half lift – inhale, as you slide your hands along your shins with a straight back, upper torso is parallel to the ground.

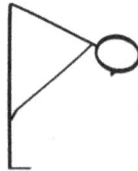

Crouching fold – exhale, as you bend down reaching your hands towards the ground; come into a tuck position, and bring your chin to your chest.

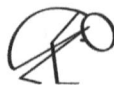

Half lift – extend your legs, as you slide your hands along your shins with a straight back, upper torso is parallel to the ground.

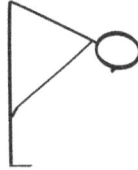

Forward fold - bend at the waist, reaching your hands towards the ground. Hang forward with a relaxed head.

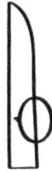

Mountain - stand tall with your arms overhead parallel to your ears, and your shoulders relaxed.

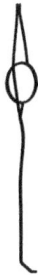

Half-moon to right - stand with your knees and feet together; squeeze your inner thighs, bring your arms up parallel to your ears and interlace your fingers. Inhale, reach up, and get taller. Exhale, and lean to the right as you squeeze your inner thighs and open your chest. Return to center position.

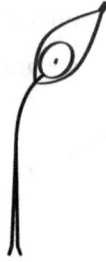

Half-moon to left - stand with your knees and feet together; squeeze your inner thighs. Inhale, reach up, and get taller. Exhale, and lean to the left as you squeeze your inner thighs and open your chest.

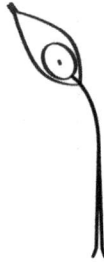

Baby backbend - lean back slightly with arms up, pressing hips forward for a slight back bend.

Hands at heart – place palms together at chest level.

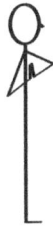

Sequence Two

Eagle pose – shift your weight to your right foot, take your left leg and wrap it over the right knee, with the toes pointing down. If you can, wrap the left foot behind the right leg, while maintaining balance. Take the left arm and cross over the right arm, bend at the elbows, and hands are back-to-back or palms touching. Bend your right knee at a 90-degree angle. Chest is open, shoulders are away from the ears. Hold for five seconds.

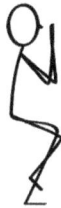

Runners lunge – unwrap your legs, bend forward, and place your hands on the ground; step your left leg back extended and straight behind you on the toes; bend your right leg at a 90-degree angle with the knee over the ankle, and the hands are on either side of your front foot.

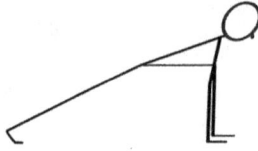

Low runners lunge - drop your left leg to ground, resting the knee and the top of the foot on the ground for an extra hip flexor stretch.

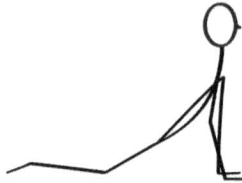

Downward dog – press back to the balls of your feet; hands on the ground shoulder-width apart; feet hip-width apart; the body is in a V; press the hips up and press the chest towards the thighs; your head should be between your arms.

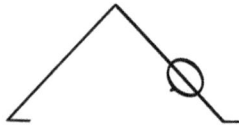

Forward fold – step both feet forward, bend at the waist and hang forward with a relaxed head.

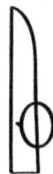

Half lift – inhale, as you slide your hands along your shins with a straight back. Upper torso comes up parallel to the ground.

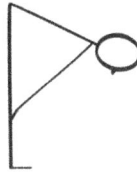

Forward fold – exhale, as you bend at the waist, reaching the hands towards the ground. Hang forward with a relaxed head.

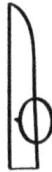

Mountain - stand tall with the arms overhead parallel to the ears, and the shoulders are relaxed.

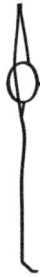

Eagle pose – shift your weight to the left foot, take your right leg and wrap it over the left knee, with toes pointing down. If you can, wrap the right foot behind the left leg while maintaining balance. Take the right arm and cross over the left arm, bend at the elbows, and hands are back-to-back or palms touching. Bend your left knee at a 90-degree angle. Chest is open, shoulders are away from the ears. Hold for five seconds.

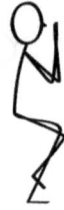

Runners lunge – unwrap your legs, bend forward and place your hands on the ground. Step your right leg back extended straight behind you with your toes on the ground. Bend your left leg at a 90-degree angle with the knee over the ankle. Hands are on either side of your foot.

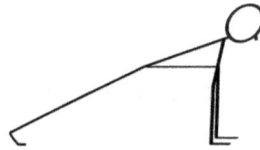

Low runners lunge - drop your right leg to ground, resting your knee and the top of your foot on the ground for an extra hip flexor stretch.

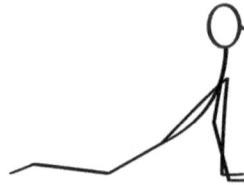

Downward dog – press back to the balls of your feet; hands on the ground shoulder-width apart; feet are hip-width apart; the body is in a V; press the hips up and press the chest towards the thighs; your head should be between your arms.

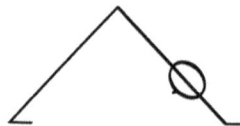

Forward fold – step both feet forward, bend at the waist, and hang forward with a relaxed head.

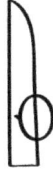

Half lift – inhale, as you slide your hands along your shins with a straight back. Upper torso comes up parallel to the ground.

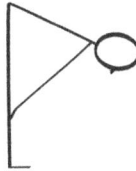

Forward fold – exhale, as you bend at the waist, and hang forward with a relaxed head.

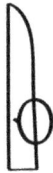

Mountain - stand tall with the arms overhead parallel to your ears, and shoulders are relaxed.

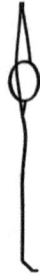

Sequence Three

Chair pose – stand with the knees and feet together; begin to bend the knees, and sit back, pretending you are sitting in an imaginary chair. Weight should be in your heels and bring your arms up parallel to your ears. Squeeze your inner thighs together and focus on the strength in your lower body.

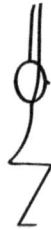

Twisting chair right – as you press your inner thighs together, bring your hands to your heart, and twist the upper body to the right as you place your left elbow on the outside of your right leg. Press into your leg for an extra twist to the right. Come back to center position with hands at the heart.

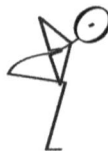

Twisting chair left – continue to press your inner thighs together and begin to twist the upper body to the left as you place your right elbow on the outside of your left leg. Press into your leg for an extra twist to the left.

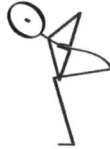

Forward fold - bend at the waist, reaching the hands towards the ground. Hang forward with a relaxed head.

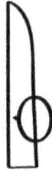

Half lift – inhale, as you slide your hands along your shins with a straight back. Upper torso comes up parallel to the ground.

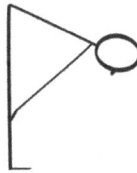

Forward fold – exhale, as you bend at the waist, and hang forward with a relaxed head.

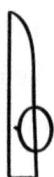

Downward dog – place your hands on the ground shoulder-width apart; step feet back hip-width apart; the body is in a V; press the hips up and press the chest towards the thighs; your head should be between your arms.

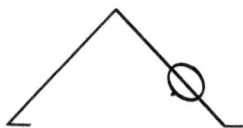

Three leg dog - lift your right leg up in the air as high as you can.

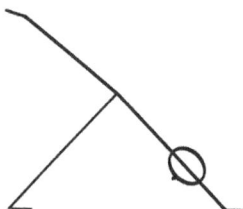

Right pigeon pose – swing the leg forward and bring your right leg to the ground sitting on your right buttock with your knee bent and your foot close to your groin. Left leg is long and extended behind you with the top of the foot resting on the ground. Square both hips, facing them forward. Hands are on the ground in front of you. Slowly begin to walk the arms and hands forward for a deeper hip stretch. If you can, place the forehead on the floor.

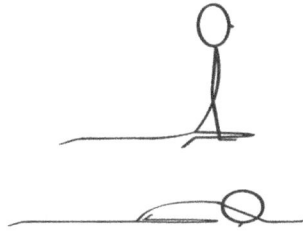

One-leg hamstring stretch - swing left leg around facing the front and have the leg straight out in front of you. Place your right ankle on your left knee. Inhale, as you reach your arms up; exhale, and begin reaching forward with your hands towards your left foot.

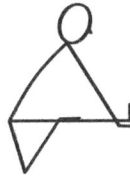

Spinal twist - bend the right leg, and place the foot flat on the floor; hug your knee into your chest, as you twist your body to the right.

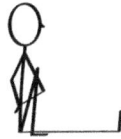

Downward dog – swing the legs behind you; place your hands on the ground shoulder-width apart; lift the knees and step your feet back hip-width apart; the body is in a V; press the hips up and press the chest towards the thighs; your head should be between your arms.

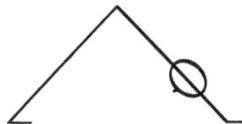

Three leg dog – lift the left leg up as high as you can, and then swing it forward.

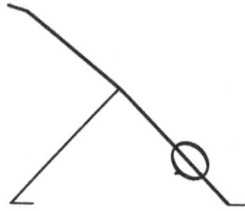

Left pigeon pose - bring the left leg to ground sitting on your left buttock with the knee bent and your foot near your groin. Right leg is extended long behind you with the top of the foot resting on the ground. Square both hips, facing them forward. Hands are on the ground in front of you. Slowly begin to walk the arms and hands forward, reaching them toward the ground for a deep hip stretch. If you can, place your forehead on the ground.

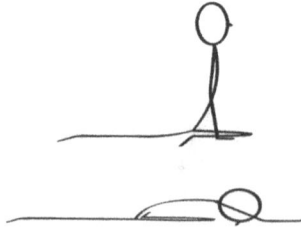

One-leg hamstring stretch - swing your right leg around facing the front and have the leg straight out in front of you. Place your left ankle on your right knee. Inhale, as you reach arms up. Exhale, as you begin to reach forward with your hands towards your right foot.

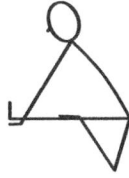

Spinal twist – bend the left leg and place the foot flat on the floor. Hug your knee into your chest and twist the body to the left.

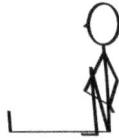

Low back stretch - lay on your back, and bring your knees into chest, rocking side to side.

Spinal twist on floor - cross the right knee over the left knee. Let your legs fall to the left on the ground for a spinal twist. Place your arms out on the floor in a T-position and move your head to the right. Come back to center.

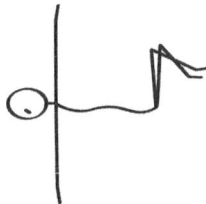

Spinal twist on floor - cross the left knee over right knee. Let the legs fall to the right for a spinal twist. Place your arms out on the floor in a T-position and move your head to the left.

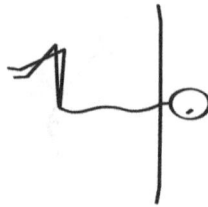

Happy baby pose – as you lay on your back, bend your knees and bring them into your belly. Grip the outsides of your feet with your hands and open your knees slightly. Position each ankle directly over the knee, so that your shins are perpendicular to the floor. Flex your feet, and gently press down on your feet. You may rock side to side as you continue to press your knees into your belly.

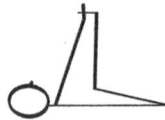

Tip of the day: Stop comparing yourself to others!

Focus of the day: Comparison to others will create a negative loop that will be difficult to erase. We have to remember that we are unique and special individuals. We do not want to be anyone else. We want to aim to be the best person we can be. Comparison to others only harms us. We should also consider who we are comparing ourselves to, because often we tend to compare ourselves to people who are in completely different situations and environments than we are. It is very hard to compare when the playing field is not even. Our focus should be trying to be the best version of ourselves that we can be!

LESSON TWELVE

Yoga

...quence One (On Back)

...w back stretch — bring your knees into your chest and rock back ...forth.

...leg low back stretch — bring the right knee into the chest and the left leg long on the ground.

...t twist — place your right arm out like a T on the ground, take ...eft hand and gently pull on your right knee, twisting it across ...ody to the left.

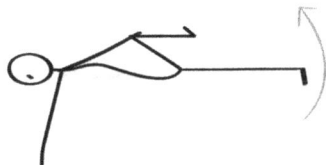

...low back stretch — bring the left knee into the chest and keep ...t leg long on the ground.

Mindful Activity: Comparison to Others

Take a moment to find a comfortable position. Allow the body to soften and relax. Let go of any tension or areas of tightness in the body. Next, bring your focus to your breath, following your inhalations fully and following your exhalations fully. Breathing should be easy and natural. Try to notice the way your body feels right now. Are there any areas that are holding on to tension or tightness? If there are, try to allow those areas of discomfort to melt away and become soft and light. Take a moment to imagine your entire body melting into the floor or melting into your chair, letting go, softening, releasing, and lengthening the entire body.

Now, I want you to think about someone you often compare yourself to. This could be a teammate, comparing yourself in regard to performance, talent, or ability. It could be a family member, a friend, or an acquaintance. Really, it could be anyone you find yourself wanting to be more like, in some way. Take a moment to bring this person to mind right now.

Now, think about what exactly it is that you want, that this person has. Is it a quality, personality trait, ability, talent, a physical attribute, or perhaps everything, an overall desire to be exactly like this person? Take a moment to pinpoint what you admire or want that the other person has. Now, I want you to consider something very important. Did you ever stop to think that this could be a learning experience for you to help improve yourself, instead of looking at it as a negative, and that you fall short in some way? Let's consider if what you desire from that person is realistic, doable, and will make you a better person because of it. When I talk about reality, what I mean is that we should not be comparing ourselves to someone who is living a completely different life than we are. Imagine this person's life and lifestyle. Is this the type of life you would want, and is this the type of person who you would want to be? Does this person have good values, morals, behaviors, and attitudes that are positive and valued? A lot of times, we tend to compare ourselves to just the outside appearance of someone and who we think they are, without truly knowing the person at all. It is important to take some time to really analyze who we are comparing ourselves to, and if this is something that can make us grow, or if it is something that will move us away from our goals. Take a moment to contemplate if your comparison to this person is a positive experience from which you can learn and become a better person, or if you realize this comparison does not serve you well at all.

Now, I want you to also consider that you are a unique, beautiful, smart, intelligent, creative individual who should be aiming to be the best possible you. You do not want or need to be someone else. You are enough the way you are. Let's focus on some self-compassion and kindness for ourselves.

Please repeat these positive affirmations to yourself now, and say them with conviction:
I am a valuable human being.
I am perfectly okay, just the way I am.
I accept myself for who I am.
I recognize that I have great talents and abilities.
I am a unique individual with a unique set of qualities.

There is no one else in this entire world that is like me.
I matter, and I am enough.
I want to be confident and proud of who I am.
I realize that I must love and respect myself first.
I want to be kinder and gentler with myself.
I recognize that I make mistakes, and that is okay.
Everyone makes mistakes.
I am important, to me.
I am proud to be me.
Slowly bring your attention back to your breathing, and an exhale. When you are ready, please open y

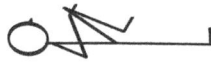

Spinal twist – place your left arm out like a T on the ground, take your right hand and gently pull on your left knee, twisting it across your body to the right. Bring back to center.

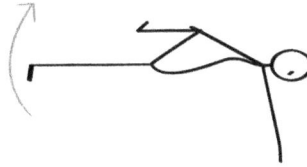

Happy baby pose – as you lay on your back, bend your knees and bring them into your belly. Grip the outsides of your feet with your hands and open your knees slightly. Position each ankle directly over the knee, so that your shins are perpendicular to the floor. Flex your feet, and gently press down on your feet. You may rock side to side as you continue to press your knees into your belly.

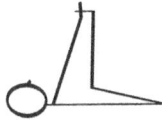

Figure four with right leg - place right ankle on left knee, place your hands behind the left knee and pull into you.

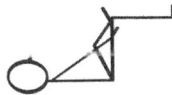

Figure four with left leg - place the left ankle on right knee, place your hands behind the right knee and pull into you.

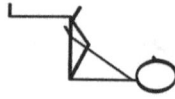

Spinal twist right - cross right knee over the left knee and let legs fall to the left for a spinal twist. Arms are out on the floor in a T-position, and your head turns to the right.

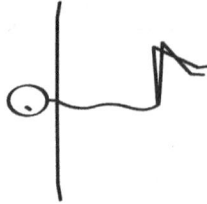

Spinal twist left – cross the left knee over the right knee and let legs fall to the right for a spinal twist. Arms are out on the floor in a T-position, and your head turns to the left.

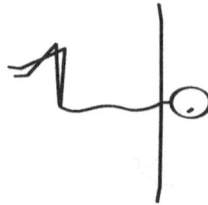

Sequence Two (Seated)

Neck rolls – bring your chin to your chest and roll your right ear to your right shoulder slowly. Bring back to center. Repeat four times.

Neck rolls – bring your chin to your chest and roll your left ear to your left shoulder slowly. Return to center. Repeat four times.

Neck turns - turn your head as far as you can to the right side, looking over your right shoulder. Then, turn your head as far as you can to the left side, looking over your left shoulder. Repeat ten times moving slowly back and forth from right side to left side.

Neck stretches – bring your chin to your chest, hold, and then back to starting position. Repeat ten times.

Side bend right – in a seated position, reach your left arm up overhead, and then lean over to the right side to stretch the left-side body.

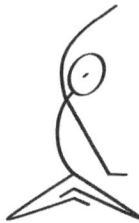

Side bend left – in a seated position, reach your right arm up overhead, and then lean over to the left side to stretch the right-side body.

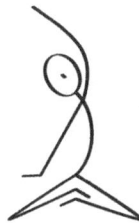

Repeat two times on each side.

Seated twist right - sit with legs crossed. Inhale, as you lift your arms up towards the ceiling, and as you exhale twist your body to the right, bringing your right hand behind you and left hand in front of you, both resting on the floor. Inhale, and bring arms back to center, parallel to your ears.

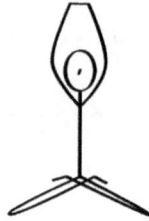

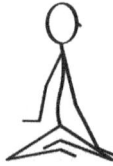

Seated twist left – As you exhale, twist your body to the left, bringing your left hand behind you and right hand in front of you, both resting on the floor.

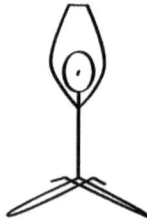

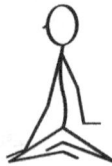

Pike stretch – sit with both legs straight in front of you. As you inhale, reach your arms up so they are parallel to your ears. As you exhale, reach for your feet with both hands. Repeat three times, inhaling as you reach up, and exhaling as you reach forward.

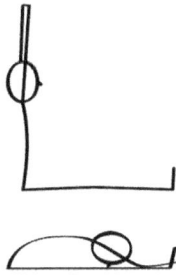

Butterfly stretch – bring the soles of feet together. As you inhale, reach up with your arms, and as you exhale, reach forward as far as you can to stretch the inner thighs.

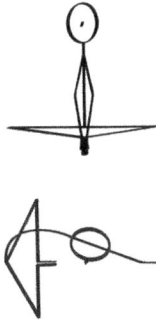

Straddle stretch – separate your legs as wide as you can on the floor. On an inhale reach up, and on an exhale reach forward as far as you can.

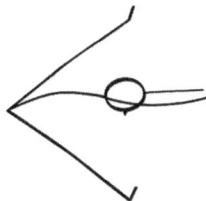

Sequence Three

Table-top – position yourself on the floor on your hands and knees, with your knees under your hips, and your hands under your shoulders.

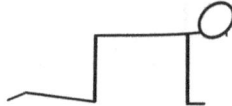

Cat cow – inhale, as the belly drops and your chin lifts. Exhale, round the back and bring your chin to your chest. Repeat five times.

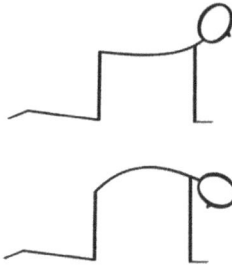

Single bow on right side - on all fours, reach the right arm forward and left leg back, pointing the toes and reaching with the fingers. Bend the leg, reach around to grab the ankle with the right hand, flex the foot, and press the foot into the hand, as you roll your shoulder back. Return to table-top position.

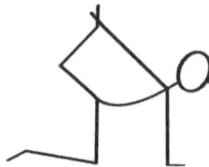

Single bow on left side - on all fours, reach the left arm forward and the right leg back, bend the leg, reach around to grab the ankle with the left hand, flex the foot, and press the foot into the hand, as you roll the shoulder back.

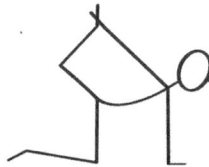

Child's pose – sit back with your buttocks on your heels. Reach the arms and hands forward on the floor, placing your forehead on the ground.

Upward dog – lay on your stomach, as you place your hands at your sides at chest level; the lower body is on the ground; press into your hands and lift upper torso and hips off the ground; arms are straight; roll the shoulders back, and look back for a slight backbend, as the tops of your feet are resting on the floor.

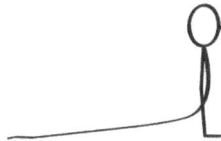

Child's pose – press back and sit with your buttocks on your heels. Reach your arms and hands forward on the floor, placing your forehead on the ground.

Upward dog – lay on your stomach, as you place hands at your sides at chest level; the lower body is on the ground; press into your hands and lift upper torso and hips off the ground; arms are straight; roll the shoulders back, and look back for a slight backbend, with the tops of the feet resting on the floor.

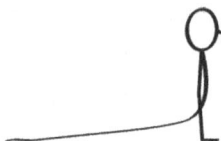

Repeat one more time (child's pose to the upward dog)

Puppy pose – come into a table-top position with the knees under the hips, and hands under the shoulders. Start leaning your buttocks towards your heels and reach your arms forward on the ground for a spine and shoulder stretch. You may rest your forehead on the ground.

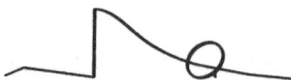

Downward dog – press back to the balls of your feet; hands on the ground shoulder-width apart; step the feet back hip-width apart; the body is in a V; press the hips up and press the chest towards the thighs; your head should be between your arms.

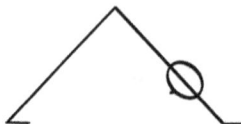

Forward fold – step your feet up, bend at the waist, and hang forward with a relaxed head.

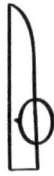

Half lift – inhale, as you slide your hands along your shins with a straight back. Upper torso comes up parallel to the ground.

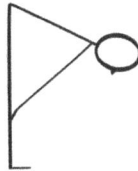

Forward fold – exhale, as you bend at the waist, and hang forward with a relaxed head.

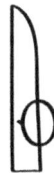

Mountain – stand tall with your arms overhead parallel to your ears, and your shoulders are relaxed.

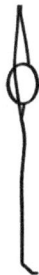

Tip of the day: Every day is a new opportunity! It does not matter what happened yesterday or what will happen tomorrow. Today is a new day, and with a new day comes new possibilities. You can change the course of your life. It is your choice.

Focus of the day: Positivity! It is so important for us to continue to focus on positive aspects of our life, positive people in our life, and positive beliefs in ourselves. Positivity breeds positivity! Do you want to be a positive person or a negative person? It can change the course of your life.

Mindful Activity: Creating A Positive Future (Mindful Exercises, 2021)

Let's begin by getting into a comfortable position. If you are seated, make sure your spine is straight but soft. Allow your shoulders to roll back and relax. If you are lying down, allow your body to elongate and lengthen. Begin by noticing your breath and take slow and steady breaths, allowing your chest to rise and fall with each breath you take. There is nothing you need to do right now, and nowhere you need to be, except in this present moment. As you breathe, allow your breath to begin to loosen areas of your body where you might be holding onto tension or stress. Notice these areas of tension, and send your breath to these tender areas, trying to loosen and soften each body part. Just relax, unwind, and allow for a calmness to sweep over your body and mind.

Now, I want you to consider this question. "What do you want your future to look like?" Take a moment to envision what you want out of your life, and what is most important to you. Notice what thoughts or images come to mind when I ask this question.

What does it mean to have a positive future for you? What does that picture look like in your mind? Create and imagine that you are living your best life, the life you want for your future.

Imagine that the future is now. What does your life look like, as you sit here and envision your positive future? I also want you to ask yourself a few more guided questions. What do you need to do in order to get there? Take a moment to consider how you would have to act or behave? Consider what type of effort or work you would need to put in? Who would be there to help guide you? Picture the answers to these questions with vivid detail. Immerse yourself in discovering the path you need to be on, in order to create your positive future. Take a moment to contemplate these questions.

Visualize one last snapshot of what your life looks like in this positive future. Know that you are the one who is calling the shots. You create your own future by the decisions you make every day. Understand that you can come back from any choice or decision that might have led you down the wrong path. You have the power to get back on the right path so that you can obtain your positive future.

Your choices matter, big and small. Each decision you make will shape your future.

Now, bring your attention back to the room and back to my voice. Allow your attention to rest with your breath. Please take a deep breath in through your nose and out through your nose. When you are ready, you may open your eyes.

LESSON THIRTEEN

Yoga

✳

Sequence One

Right side

Warrior 1 – step your right leg forward and bend your right leg at a 90-degree angle. Your left leg is straight behind you, with the feet around four feet apart. Make sure your left foot is turned out slightly. Square your hips, so that they face forward, and reach your arms up parallel to your ears. Keep your right knee over your right ankle.

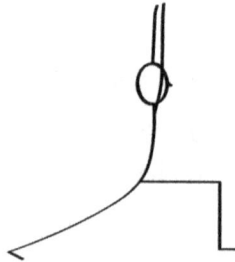

Warrior 2- lower your arms, as you turn your upper body to the left. Your arms are parallel to the floor, reaching out with the fingers. Right arm is forward and left arm is back. Bend your front leg at a 90-degree angle, and your back leg stays firm and straight. Gaze over your front middle finger.

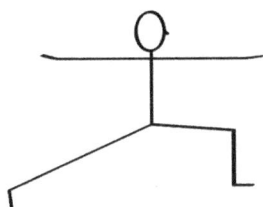

Warrior 3 – shift your weight to your right foot. Lift your left leg up so that it is parallel to the floor, with the big toe facing down. Press out with your heel. Hands are at your sides as you look forward and balance.

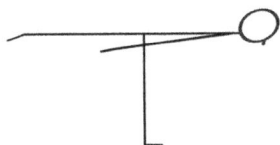

Pyramid pose- place left foot back on the ground about two-three feet from your right foot. Square your hips, so that they face forward. Both feet should be facing forward as well. As you inhale, reach your arms up parallel to your ears. As you exhale, lean forward, bending from the waist over your front leg. Reach your hands for either your shin or the floor for a hamstring stretch. Press back with your front leg in order to feel a deeper stretch.

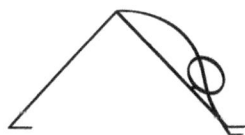

Right runners lunge – place your hands on the ground on either side of your right foot. Step your left leg back extended and firm behind you, with the toes resting on the ground. Bend your right leg at a 90-

degree angle, with the right knee over the right ankle. Sink into your hip.

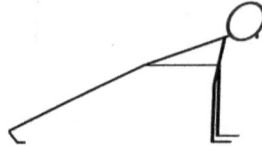

Lunge with a twist - bring your left hand to the inside of the right foot and lift your right arm up to the ceiling as you open your chest. Eyes follow the rising hand. Place your hand back.

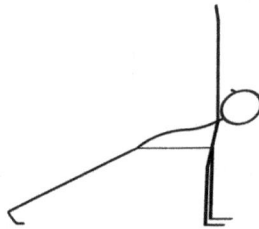

High plank – step the right leg back; hands under the shoulders; feet hip-width apart; core is tight; and shoulders are rolled back.

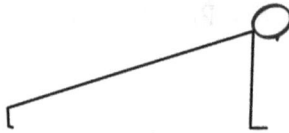

Lower yourself to the ground, leading with the chest and keeping your arms in, close to the body.

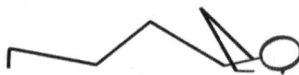

Upward dog - place hands at your sides at chest level with the lower body on the ground; press into your hands and lift upper torso and hips off the ground; arms are straight; roll the shoulders back, and look back for a slight backbend, with the tops of the feet resting on the floor.

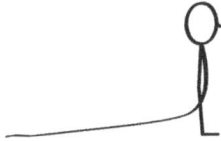

Downward dog – press back onto the balls of your feet; hands on the ground shoulder-width apart; feet are hip-width apart; the body is in a V; press the hips up and press the chest towards the thighs; your head should be between your arms.

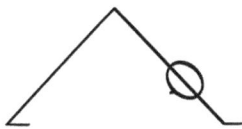

Forward fold – step feet up, and bend at the waist, reaching your arms and hands towards the ground. Hang forward with a relaxed head.

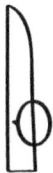

Half lift – inhale, as you slide your hands along your shins with a straight back. Upper torso comes up parallel to the ground.

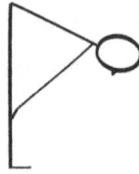

Forward fold – exhale, as you bend at the waist, and hang forward with a relaxed head.

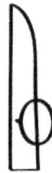

Mountain - stand tall with the arms overhead parallel to the ears, and the shoulders are relaxed.

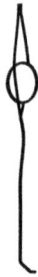

Repeat sequence on the left side starting with warrior 1 (Follow below)

Warrior 1 – step your left leg forward and bend your left leg at a 90-degree angle. Your right leg is straight behind you, with the feet around four feet apart. Make sure your right foot is turned out slightly. Square your hips, so that they face forward, and reach your arms up parallel to your ears. Keep your left knee over your left ankle.

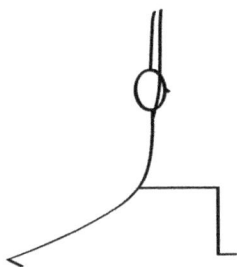

Warrior 2 – lower your arms, as you turn your upper body to the right. Your arms are parallel to the floor, reaching out with the fingers. Left arm is forward and right arm is back. Bend your front leg at a 90-degree angle, and your back leg stays firm and straight. Gaze over your front middle finger.

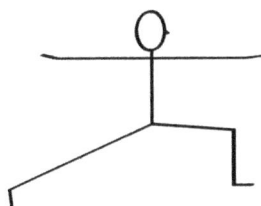

Warrior 3 – shift your weight to your left foot. Lift your right leg up so that it is parallel to the floor, with the big toe facing down. Press out with your heel. Hands are at your sides as you look forward and balance.

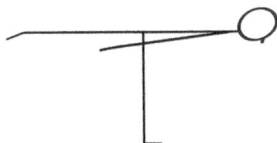

Pyramid - place the right foot back on the ground about two-three feet from your left foot. Square your hips, so that they face forward. Both feet should be facing forward as well. As you inhale, reach your arms up parallel to your ears. As you exhale, lean forward, bending from the waist over your front leg. Reach your hands for either your shin or the floor for a hamstring stretch. Press back with your front leg in order to feel a deeper stretch.

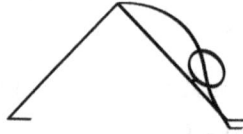

Left runners lunge – place your hands on the ground on either side of your left foot. Step your right leg back extended and firm behind you, with the toes resting on the ground. Bend your left leg at a 90-degree angle, with the left knee over the left ankle. Sink into your hip.

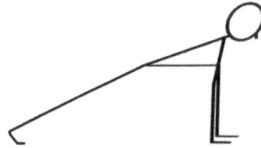

Lunge with a twist - bring your right hand to the inside of the left foot and lift your left arm up to the ceiling as you open your chest.

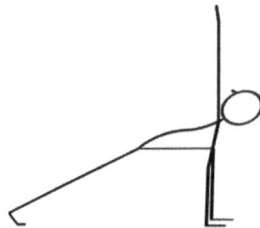

High plank - step the left leg back; hands under the shoulders; feet are hip-width apart; core is tight; and the shoulders are rolled back.

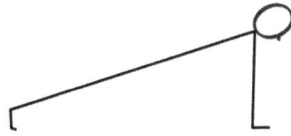

Lower yourself to the ground, leading with the chest and keeping your arms in, close to the body.

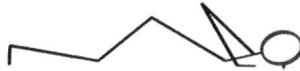

Upward dog - place hands at your sides at chest level with the lower body on the ground; press into your hands and lift upper torso and hips off the ground; arms are straight; roll the shoulders back, and look back for a slight backbend, with the tops of the feet on the floor.

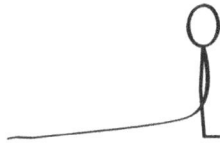

Downward dog – press back onto the balls of your feet; hands on the ground shoulder-width apart; feet are hip-width apart; the body is in a V; press the hips up and press the chest towards the thighs; your head should be between your arms.

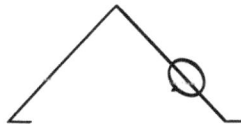

Forward fold - step feet up, bend at the waist, and hang forward with a relaxed head.

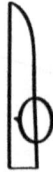

Half lift- inhale, as you slide your hands along your shins with a straight back. Upper torso comes up parallel to the ground.

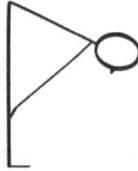

Forward fold – exhale, as you bend at the waist, and hang forward with a relaxed head.

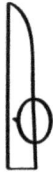

Mountain - stand tall with the arms overhead parallel to the ears, and the shoulders are relaxed.

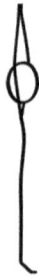

Sequence Two

Chair pose – stand with the knees and feet together, squeezing your inner thighs, bend your knees, and sit back as if you are sitting in an imaginary chair, with the weight on your heels. Raise your arms up so that they are parallel to your ears.

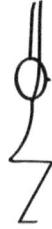

Twisting chair- bring your hands to the heart with your palms together. Twist your upper torso to the right and place your left elbow to the outside of your right knee. Press into your upper leg for an extra twist. Come back to center with palms together.

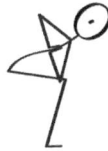

Twisting chair -twist your upper torso to the left and place your right elbow to the outside of your left knee. Press into your upper leg for an extra twist. Come back to center with palms together.

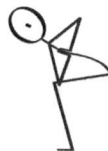

Forward fold - bend at the waist, reaching the hands towards the ground. Hang forward with a relaxed head.

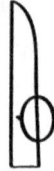

Wide leg forward fold - walk your feet wide, your toes should face forward. Reach your hands towards the ground in the center for an inner thigh stretch.

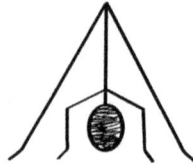

Right leg stretch - walk your hands to the right ankle, and hold for three breaths. Come back to center.

Left leg stretch - walk your hands to the left ankle, and hold for three breaths. Come back to center.

Shifting weight – with the legs wide, keep your hands in the center, and shift your weight to the balls of your feet, and then back to your heels, lifting the toes. Repeat shifting your weight back and forth six times.

Forward fold – step feet together, reach your hands towards the ground. Hang forward with a relaxed head.

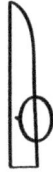

Mountain - stand tall with the arms overhead parallel to your ears, and the shoulders are relaxed.

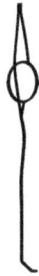

Sequence Three (Balance)

Tree pose – shift your weight to your left foot and place your right foot either on the lower shin or upper thigh of the left leg; knee is parallel to the ground, and hands come to the heart with palms together or bring your arms overhead for a balance. Hold for ten seconds.

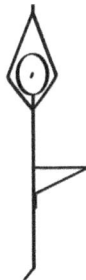

Dancer's Pose – lift your right leg behind you, and with your right hand, grab the top of the foot or ankle. Stretch your left arm up parallel to your ear, and begin to lean forward, pressing your foot into your hand, as you reach out and lower your left arm until it is parallel with the ground. This is a balance pose. Hold for ten seconds.

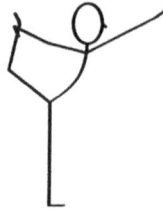

Warrior 3 - release the foot and bring the right leg parallel to the floor with the big toe facing the ground, and arms are at your sides. Hold for ten seconds.

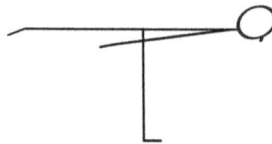

Repeat sequence on other side (follow below)

Tree pose – shift your weight to your right foot, place your left foot either on the lower shin or upper thigh of the right leg; knee is parallel to the ground, and hands come to the heart or bring your arms overhead for a balance. Hold for ten seconds.

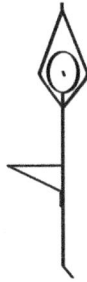

Dancer's Pose – lift your left leg behind you, and with your left hand, grab the top of the foot or the ankle. Stretch your right arm up parallel to your ear, and begin to lean forward, pressing your foot into your hand, as you reach out and lower your right arm until it is parallel with the ground. This is a balance pose. Hold for ten seconds.

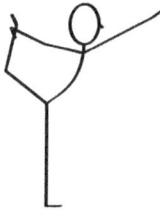

Warrior 3 - release the foot and bring the left leg parallel to the floor with the big toe facing the ground, and arms are at your sides. Hold for ten seconds. Place foot back on the ground.

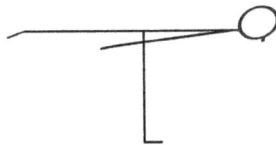

Forward fold - bend at the waist, reaching your hands towards the ground. Hang forward with a relaxed head.

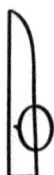

Rocking - grab the elbows, and gently rock side to side loosening the low back.

Mountain - stand tall with your arms overhead parallel to your ears, and the shoulders are relaxed.

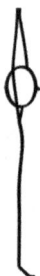

Tip of the day: Face your emotions and face your fears head-on!

Focus of the day: Feeling our emotions is a natural part of life. Emotions are here for a reason, and they are here to teach us and inform us of what is going on in our life. By pushing emotions away, we get further from the truth. We create a build-up of stress and anxiety that mounts up very rapidly. This stress and anxiety can cause us to get physically ill and not perform at our best. The answer is to accept what is, and allow yourself to feel sadness, pain, hurt, guilt, or fear. These are usually the emotions that we push away, because they are uncomfortable. We need to learn that by being uncomfortable, we can make positive changes. It is healthy and natural to allow ourselves to feel all emotions, so they do not have control or power over us. When we shut them down, they begin to take over in the form of anxiety, stress, depression, anger, and frustration.

Mindful Activity: Progressive Muscle Relaxation

For this exercise, we will be laying down, so make yourself comfortable as you lay down on your back with your palms facing up. Close your eyes and allow your focus to be with your breathing. As you inhale, feel your chest rise, and as you exhale, feel your chest lower. Continue to breathe normally and naturally, allowing fresh oxygen to circulate throughout your whole body.

The goal of this practice is for you to feel the difference between tightness and tenseness in your body and to allow for full release and softness. We will begin with our right leg. Please scrunch up the toes of your right foot, and tense up your entire foot, squeeze your buttocks and your thigh as tightly as you can. Keep squeezing and holding tension from your right hip down to your toes. It should feel uncomfortable and awkward; keep squeezing, and now let go. Release your entire right leg. Let your leg fall where it falls. Draw an imaginary line from your right hip all the way down to your toes, letting all your muscles elongate and lengthen. Now, bring your attention to your entire left leg, from your hip to your toes. Tighten and squeeze your toes, buttocks, and thigh as tightly as you can; keep squeezing and tensing, and then let it all go. Allow your left leg to completely relax and fall where it falls. Draw an imaginary line from your left hip all the way down to your toes, letting all your muscles soften and release.

Now, from your hips to your toes, you should feel completely relaxed and soft.

Bring your attention to your belly. Tense up your tummy like you were doing a crunch. Keep squeezing and tightening your tummy. Now, let it go and feel how relaxed your tummy feels.

Bring your focus to your right arm. Starting from your shoulder to your fingers, tense up your right arm by making a fist with your hand, tightening up your bicep, triceps, and forearm. Continue to squeeze and create tension here. Now, allow your arm to completely let go and relax. Draw an imaginary line from your right shoulder all the way down to your fingers, allowing every muscle fiber in your arm to relax.

Next, tense up your left arm by making a fist, squeezing your bicep, triceps, and forearm tightly. Keep squeezing, and now let it all go. Draw an imaginary line from the top of your left shoulder all the way down to your fingers, allowing your muscles to melt.

Next, bring your focus to your shoulders. Bring your shoulders up to your ears, and squeeze your shoulders tightly. Keep them lifted and tense. Now, drop your shoulders as far away from your ears as possible, allowing them to soften.

Bring your attention to the muscles in your face. You can scrunch up your face for a moment and squeeze your eyelids tightly. Then, allow the muscles of your face to release and soften. Your entire body should be completely at peace, calm, relaxed, and melting into the floor.

Notice your entire body lying here on the floor, feeling heavy and warm, full of tranquility. Take a moment to enjoy this state of complete peacefulness and relaxation.

When you are ready, you can slowly begin to wiggle your toes and fingers, bringing life back into the body. You may open your eyes.

LESSON FOURTEEN

Yoga

Sequence One

Child's pose – sit with your buttocks on your heels, and reach your arms forward on the floor, placing your forehead on the ground.

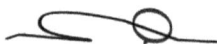

Thread the needle (shoulder stretch) - thread the right arm under the left arm, pressing the right shoulder and the right ear to the ground. Come back to center.

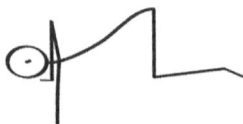

Thread the needle (shoulder stretch) - thread the left arm under the right arm, pressing the left shoulder and the left ear to the ground. Come back to center.

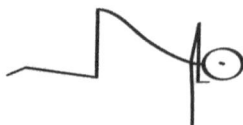

Cat cow – come into a table-top position, with the hands under the shoulders, and the knees under the hips. Inhale, as you drop the belly and lift your chin. Exhale, as you round your back and bring your chin to your chest.

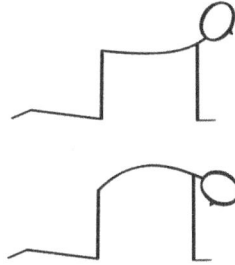

Child's pose – sit back with your buttocks on your heels. Reach the hands forward, placing your forehead on the ground.

Cat cow – get into a table-top position. Inhale, as you drop the belly and lift your chin. Exhale, as you round your back and bring your chin to your chest.

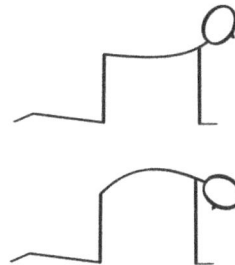

Sequence Two

Downward dog – press back onto the balls of your feet; hands on the ground shoulder-width apart; feet are hip-width apart; the body is in a V; press the hips up and press the chest towards the thighs; your head should be between your arms.

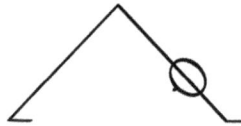

Walk the dog – pedal the right and left heels towards the ground for a calf stretch.

Three leg dog - lift the right leg high into the air, and then swing it through to place the right buttocks on the ground.

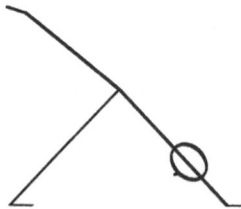

Pigeon pose - sit on the right buttocks with the knee bent, and your foot near your groin. Your left leg is extended, straight behind you on the floor with the top of the foot resting on the ground. Hands are flat on the floor in front of you. When you are ready, lean forward and reach your hands out as far as you can, dropping your forehead to the ground.

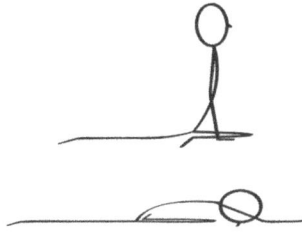

Downward dog – press back onto the balls of your feet; hands on the ground shoulder-width apart; feet are hip-width apart; the body is in a V; press the hips up and press the chest towards the thighs; your head should be between your arms.

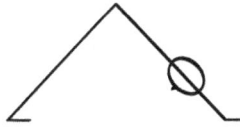

Three leg dog - lift the left leg high into the air, and then swing it through to place your left buttocks on the ground.

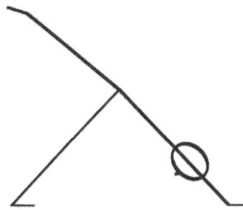

Pigeon pose – sit on the left buttocks with the knee bent, and your foot near your groin. Your right leg is extended, straight behind you on the floor with the top of your foot resting on the ground. Hands are flat on the floor in front of you. When you are ready, lean forward, and reach your hands out as far as you can, dropping your forehead to the ground.

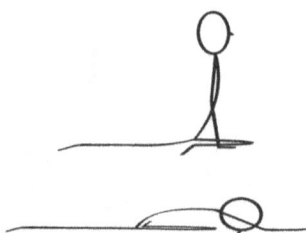

Downward dog – press back onto the balls of your feet; hands on the ground shoulder-width apart; feet are hip-width apart; the body is in a V; press the hips up and press the chest towards the thighs; your head should be between your arms.

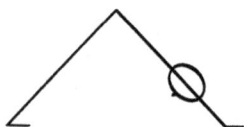

Forward fold – step feet up, bend at the waist, and hang forward with a relaxed head.

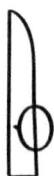

Half lift – inhale, as you slide your hands along your shins with a straight back. Upper torso comes up parallel to the ground.

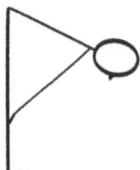

Forward fold – exhale, as you bend at the waist, and hang forward with a relaxed head.

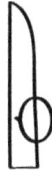

Chair pose – stand with your knees and feet together. Squeeze your inner thighs together, as you sit back in an imaginary chair, with your weight on your heels, and your arms up parallel to your ears.

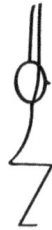

Forward fold - bend at the waist, reaching your hands towards the ground. Hang forward with a relaxed head.

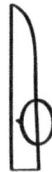

Half lift – inhale, as you slide your hands along your shins with a straight back. Upper torso comes up parallel to the ground.

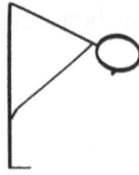

Forward fold – exhale, as you bend at the waist, and hang forward with a relaxed head.

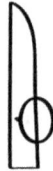

Chair pose – stand with your knees and feet together. Squeeze your inner thighs together, as you sit back in an imaginary chair, with your weight on your heels, and your arms up parallel to your ears.

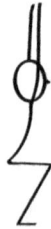

Forward fold - bend at the waist, reaching your hands towards the ground. Hang forward with a relaxed head.

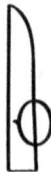

Half lift – inhale, as you slide your hands along your shins with a straight back. Upper torso comes up parallel to the ground.

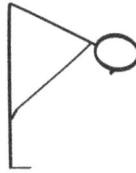

Forward fold – exhale, as you bend at the waist, and hang forward with a relaxed head.

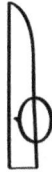

Runners lunge – place your hands on the ground on either side of your left foot. Step your right leg back extended and firm behind you, resting on the toes. Your left leg is bent at a 90-degree angle, with your knee over your ankle.

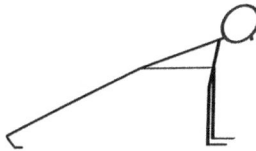

Low runners lunge - drop your right leg to the ground, resting your knee and the top of the foot on the floor. Press your hip to the floor.

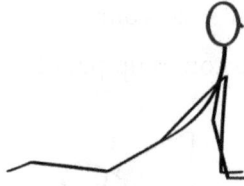

Low crescent lunge – stay in the low runners lunge and lift your arms up parallel to your ears. Continue to press your right hip into the ground.

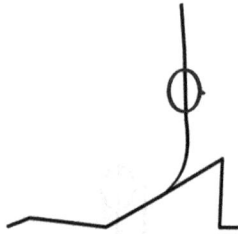

Twist - bring your hands to your heart with your palms together. Twist your upper body to the left, bringing your right elbow on the outside of the left knee. Press your elbow into your knee for an extra twist.

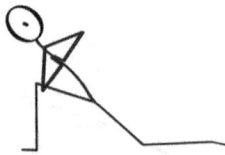

Runners lunge – place your hands back on the ground on either side of your left foot, and lift the back leg off the ground, to rest on the toes.

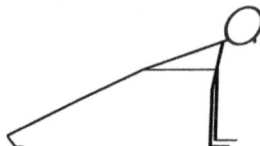

Forward fold – step your foot up, so that both feet are together. Bend at the waist, reaching the hands towards the floor. Hang forward with a relaxed head.

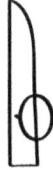

Runners lunge – place your hands on the ground on either side of your right foot. Step your left leg back extended and long behind you, resting on the toes. Your right leg is bent at a 90-degree angle with the knee over the ankle.

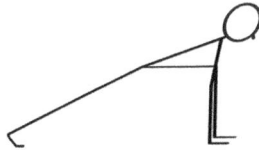

Low runners lunge - drop your left leg to the ground, resting the knee and the top of your foot on the floor. Press your hip to the floor.

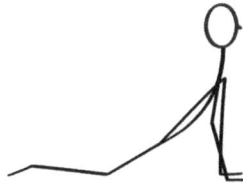

Low crescent lunge – stay in a low runners lunge, and lift your arms up parallel to your ears.

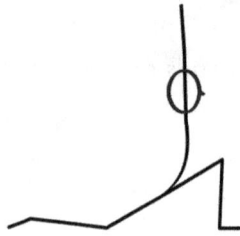

Twist -bring your hands to your heart with the palms together. Twist your upper body to the right, bringing your left elbow on the outside of the right knee. Press your elbow into your knee for an extra twist.

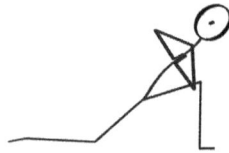

Runners lunge - place your hands back on the ground on either side of your right foot, and lift the back leg off the ground, resting on the toes.

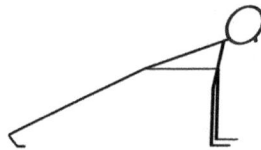

Forward fold - step foot up so that both feet are together. Bend at the waist and hang forward with a relaxed head.

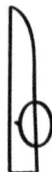

Half lift – inhale, as you slide your hands along your shins with a straight back. Upper torso comes up parallel to the ground.

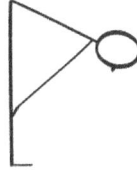

Forward fold – exhale, as you bend at the waist, and hang forward with a relaxed head.

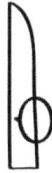

Wide leg forward fold – separate your feet as wide as you can, with your toes pointing forward. Place your hands on the ground in front of you and press back onto your heels.

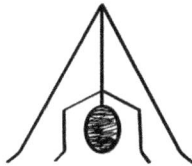

Twist right – place your left hand on the ground directly under your face, and twist the upper body to the right, lifting your right arm up towards the ceiling. Try not to sway or move your hips. Come back to center.

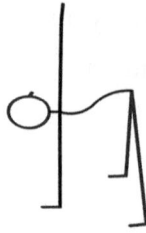

Twist left – place your right hand on the ground directly under your face, and twist the upper body to the left, lifting your left arm up towards the ceiling, trying not to sway or move the hips.

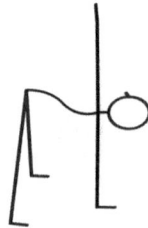

Chest stretch - interlace your fingers behind you, adding a chest stretch to the pose. When you are ready, lift your arms up as high as you can. Return your hands to center.

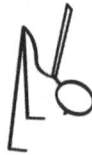

Low yoga squat – bend your knees and squat down. Place your hands at the heart, with the palms together. Place your elbows on your inner thighs. Press your elbows into your inner thighs; feet are flat on the floor or the heels are raised. This is an inner thigh stretch.

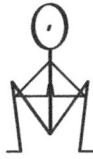

Forward fold – stand up and bring the feet together. Bend at the waist, reaching the hands towards the ground. Hang forward with a relaxed head.

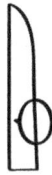

Child's pose – sit with your buttocks on your heels. Reach your hands forward, placing your forehead on the ground.

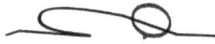

Sequence Three (Seated Position)

Reclined pigeon (figure four stretch) – cross the right ankle over the left knee, with the left foot flat on the floor. Sit up tall with your chest open, shoulders rolled back, and your hands behind you resting on the floor shoulder-width apart.

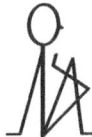

Spinal twist - straighten your left leg long on the ground, bend your right knee into your chest, hug your knee, and twist your upper body to the right.

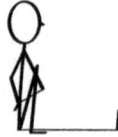

Spinal twist lying down - lay down and place your left hand on your right knee, pressing on your right knee and crossing it over the body to the left. Right arm is extended on the ground in a T-position. Your head is turned to face the right.

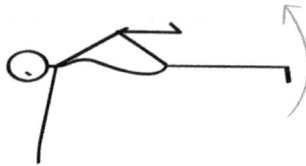

Knees into the chest – bring both knees into your chest and rock side to side to loosen the low back.

Rolling like a ball - rock yourself back and forth in a tuck position and come up to a seated position.

Reclined pigeon (figure four stretch) - cross the left ankle over the right knee, with the right foot flat on the floor. Sit up tall with your chest open, shoulders rolled back, and your hands behind you resting on the floor shoulder-width apart.

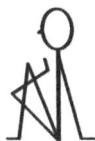

Spinal twist - straighten your right leg long on the ground, bend your left knee into your chest, hug your knee, and twist your upper body to the left.

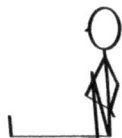

Spinal twist lying down - lay down and place your right hand on your left knee, pressing on your left knee and crossing it over the body to right. Left arm is extended on the ground in a T-position. Your head turns to the left.

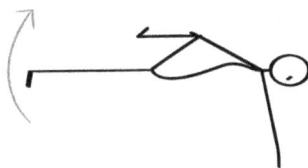

Knees into the chest - bring both knees into your chest and rock side to side to loosen the low back.

Happy baby pose – lay on your back, bend your knees and bring them into your belly. Grip the outsides of your feet with your hands and open your knees slightly. Position each ankle directly over the knee, so that your shins are perpendicular to the floor. Flex your feet, and gently press down on your feet. You may rock side to side as you continue to press your knees into your belly.

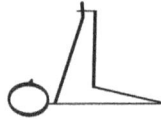

Full body stretch – straighten your legs and reach your arms overhead for a full body stretch.

Tip of the day: Burdick (2014) talks about knowing that you have the power to change your viewing channel anytime you want to. Your mind determines your mood, and you do not have to stay on the same bad channel in your mind all the time. Remember, a thought causes an emotion and an emotion causes a reaction.

Focus of the day: The mind is a very powerful tool. Our thoughts determine if we are in a good mood or a bad mood. Have you ever been completely fine one minute, and then all of a sudden, you have a thought, and it completely changes your mood from positive to negative? It is important to begin paying attention to the thoughts we have every day, so that we can recognize when we are getting off track and heading down a dark path. We can change that path.

Mindful Activity: Labeling Thoughts & Watching Them Drift Away as Clouds

Let's begin by getting into a comfortable position and allowing our bodies to relax and unwind. Take a moment to settle in, and just notice how you are feeling at this exact moment in time. We start out by noticing what thoughts are circling around in our heads. No need to change them; just notice where your mind wants to go right now. Then, we take notice of our body and how that is feeling at this very moment in time. Are we tight or tense anywhere, or are we relaxed and soft? Just notice.

Next, we tune into our breath and notice how we are breathing at this moment in time. Is our breathing shallow or perhaps a bit deeper right now? In order for us to be able to make sense of why we feel the way we do sometimes, we need to tune into our thoughts. These very thoughts are what cause us to feel emotions.

For this visualization, I want you to become aware of any thoughts that you are having. Each time you have a thought, I want you to note whether it is positive, negative, or neutral. You can also get into more detail if you want, by labeling the thought as planning, fantasizing, worrying, having memories, or judging yourself. Take a moment to notice what thoughts pop up for you, and try to give them appropriate labels, if you can.

After you label the thought, try to bring your attention back to each inhale and exhale, until you have another thought to label. Remember, labeling is really important in order to understand why we feel the way we do. Do your best to label your thoughts as planning, fantasizing, worrying, having memories, or judging. If this is too difficult, then just note if the thought is positive, negative, or neutral. (Pause)

Your mind might be swirling around with so many thoughts that you are finding it difficult to track, and that is okay if that is what is happening. Just allow your mind to go and do the best you can. You may also be sitting here thinking things like, this is silly, I can't do this, or this is stupid. This is also okay, if that is what is happening. Just try to put the label on the thought and bring your attention back to your breathing.

Now, I want you to imagine that you are sitting outside somewhere on the most beautiful sunny day. You could be sitting near the water, on a bench, or lying on a blanket in a field. It is your choice where you want to visualize yourself on this beautiful day. Take a moment to picture where you are.

Now, each time you have a thought, I want you to imagine that you are looking up at the sky, noticing the fluffy white clouds passing by. Now, imagine placing each thought on a cloud in the sky and watch it float away. For each and every thought, place it on the fluffy white cloud and watch it drift far away from you. You can return your attention to the sunny blue sky after your thought has passed away. Continue to do this for a few moments, and just notice how this is for you. (Pause)

Now, I want you to repeat these statements to yourself:

I am always in control of my thoughts.

I have the power to change and challenge my thoughts.

I do not have to believe my thoughts.

My thoughts are not my reality.

Repeat each statement one more time

Bring your attention to your breathing again, following each inhalation and each exhalation. When you are ready, you may open your eyes.

LESSON FIFTEEN

Yoga

❋

Sequence One (On the back)

Knees into chest - bring both knees into chest and rock side to side.

Spinal twist right– laying on your back, with knees into chest, allow knees to fall to the right for a twist. Place arms on the ground in a T-position. Bring knees back to center.

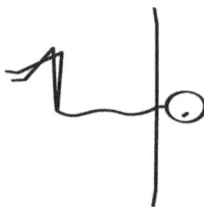

Spinal twist left- allow knees to fall to the left for a twist. Bring them back to center.

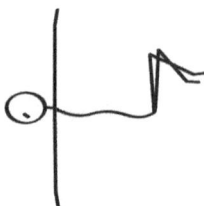

One-leg back stretch – hug your right knee into your chest, and let the left leg stay on the floor long and extended.

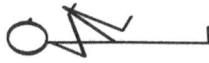

Hamstring stretch - straighten the right leg to the ceiling, place your hands behind your knee, or reach for your toes, and gently press your leg toward you.

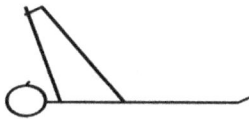

One-leg stretch – hug the left knee into your chest and let the right leg rest on the floor extended and straight.

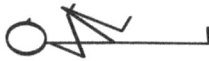

Hamstring stretch – straighten the left leg up towards the ceiling, place your hands behind your knee, or reach for your toes, and gently press the leg toward you.

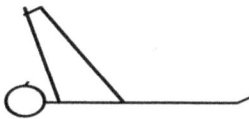

Double hamstring stretch – straighten both legs towards the ceiling, placing your hands behind your knees, or reach for your feet, and gently press your legs towards you.

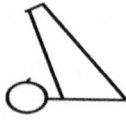

Rolling like a ball – bend your knees into your chest, staying in a tuck position, rock forward and back, keeping your core tight. Arms should be at your sides and use your stomach muscles to rock yourself to a seated position, balancing on the buttocks. Repeat the rolling like a ball five times.

Shoulder stand -as you roll back on your fifth time, bring your hands to your hips immediately as you rest your upper arms on the ground, and raise your legs straight towards the celling. You are holding your body upright. Keep your legs together and hold yourself up for five breaths.

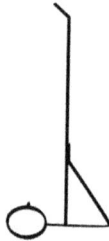

Single cow pose (crossed legs on back)- laying on your back, cross your right knee over your left knee, bring the feet close to your buttocks, and grab your ankles with your hands. Pull them into you.

Single cow pose (crossed legs on back) – laying on your back, cross your left knee over your right knee, bring the feet close to your buttocks, and grab your ankles with your hands. Pull them into you.

Shoulder bridge - lay on your back with your knees bent, and feet flat on the floor aligned under your knees. Place your arms under your body and interlace your fingers. Roll your shoulders back, and lift your lower body off the ground, as you press into your feet. Lift your hips up as high as you can. Hold for five breaths. Lower your hips to the ground.

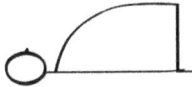

Happy baby pose – lay on your back, bend your knees and bring them into your belly. Grip the outsides of your feet with your hands and open your knees slightly. Position each ankle directly over the knee, so that your shins are perpendicular to the floor. Flex your feet, and gently press down on your feet. You may rock side to side as you continue to press your knees into your belly.

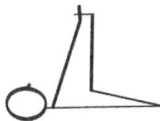

Table-top – position yourself on the floor on your hands and knees, with your knees under your hips, and your hands under your shoulders.

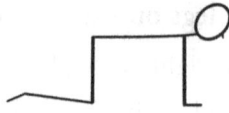

Cat cow – inhale, as you drop the belly and lift the chin. Exhale, as you round your back and bring your chin to your chest. Repeat five times.

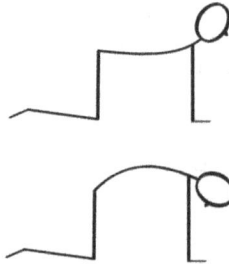

Sequence Two

Right runners lunge – bring your right leg forward at a 90-degree angle, with the knee and ankle aligned. Hands are on either side of your right foot. Step the left leg back, extended straight and firm behind you with the toes on the ground.

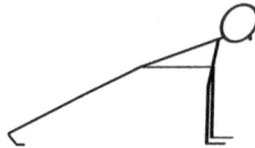

Low runners lunge - drop your left leg to the ground, resting the knee and the top of the foot on the floor. Press your hip to the floor.

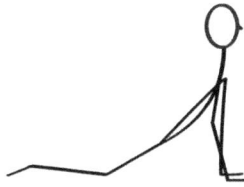

Split leg stretch - sit back with your buttocks on your left heel and straighten the right leg out in front of you. Inhale, reaching your arms up, parallel to the ears. As you exhale, lean forward and try to touch your toes with your hands.

Pigeon pose - bend your right leg, so that your foot is near your groin and you are resting on your right buttocks. Extend your left leg straight behind you, with your left hip pressing towards the floor, and the top of your foot resting on the ground. Sit up tall, with your hands flat on the floor in front of you. Begin to lower yourself towards the ground, reaching your arms and hands forward as far as you can, and bring your forehead to the ground.

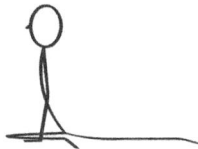

Quad stretch – sit up, hands on the ground, reach around and grab your left ankle with your left hand, face forward, and pull the foot towards your buttocks for a quad stretch.

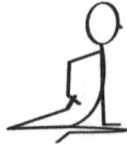

Repeat sequence on the left side (follow below)

Left runners lunge – step the left leg forward and bend it at a 90-degree angle, with the knee and ankle aligned. Hands are on either side of your left foot. Step right leg back, extended straight behind you with your toes resting on the floor.

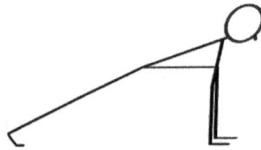

Low runners lunge - drop your right leg to the ground, resting the knee and top of the foot on the floor. Press your hip to the floor.

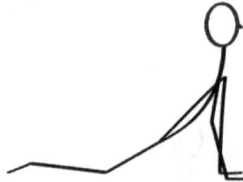

Split leg stretch - sit back with your buttocks on your right heel and straighten the left leg out in front of you. Inhale, as you reach your arms up, parallel to your ears. As you exhale, begin to lean forward and try to touch your toes with your hands.

Pigeon pose - bend your left leg, so that your foot is near your groin and you are resting on your left buttocks. Extend your right leg straight behind you, with your right hip pressing towards the floor. Sit up tall with your hands on the ground in front of you. Begin to reach your arms and hands forward on the floor as far as you can and bring your forehead to the ground.

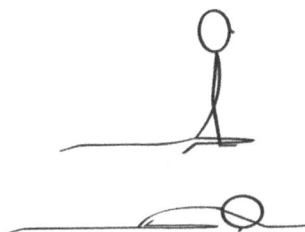

Quad stretch – sit up, place your hands on the ground in front of you. Reach around and grab your right ankle with your right hand, face forward, and gently pull the foot towards your buttocks for a quad stretch.

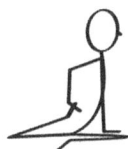

Sequence Three

Camel back bend – start by sitting with your buttocks on your heels. Lift your buttocks off your heels, make sure your shins are on the floor, knees are under your hips, place your hands on your low back, press your hips forward, and begin to backbend. Go to a place that is comfortable for you.

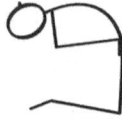

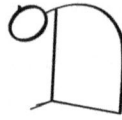

Half camel – if you can, lean back and grab your left ankle with your left hand, as you swing your right arm up, reaching back.

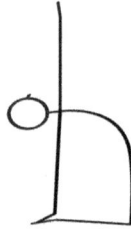

Half camel – come back to center, and then lean back and grab your right ankle with your right hand as you swing your left arm up, reaching back.

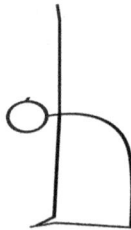

Repeat two more times on each side flowing between right and left half-camel.

Wide child's pose -sit with your buttocks on your heels, and your knees wide. Reach your hands out in front of you as far as you can.

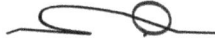

Full body stretch – lay down on your back, straighten your legs on the floor, and reach with the toes. Reach your arms overhead for a full body stretch, reaching with the fingers.

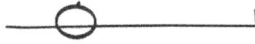

Tip of the day: Schedule ME time each day. This is a time when you allow yourself to relax and do something you truly enjoy. It is essential to make time for yourself every day, because you MATTER.

Focus of the day: Learning to have balance in your life. Balance is finding the right amount of time to spend doing things you enjoy, and doing things you need to do to be successful (school/work). You never want to be too one-sided with this. You will be the best you and the most effective you when you have found the perfect balance in life, so you don't get too stressed out.

Mindful Activity: Heightening Awareness

Let's begin by finding a comfortable, mindful body position. This means we are seated comfortably, the spine is straight but soft, and shoulders are away from our ears. The body is comfortable and able to stay aware. Take a moment to notice if there are any sounds in the room. Each time you hear a sound, take a moment to really focus on that one sound. When you hear another sound, bring your attention to the new sound, and see if you can also stay with that one sound for a moment. Allow any sounds to come into your awareness. The sounds might be very easy to hear and loud, or the sounds could be very subtle and soft. Just see how many sounds you notice. These sounds could be sounds outside the body, or they could be sounds that your own body is making that you notice. For instance, you may hear your tummy growl, or maybe you could hear your breathing as you breathe in and out of your nose. Simply become aware of sound.

Next, switch your awareness to your body. Notice how your body feels right now. Where is the first place which grabs your attention, when you are trying to become aware of your body? Are you noticing any tightness, soreness, tension anywhere in the body today? Do you notice any areas that are relaxed and feel good today? Can you notice any changes in temperature in your body? Are any body parts warmer or cooler than the others? Just notice and be with whatever is. Can you feel your clothes against your body?

Next, we switch our awareness to our breathing. Become focused on each breath you take, and follow the flow of your breathing as you inhale and exhale. Where are you noticing your breath the most today? Can you feel the breath in the nostrils, chest, or belly? Can you notice the temperature change of the air coming in and the air moving out of your nostrils? Take a moment to follow each breath fully, knowing that you are sending fresh oxygen to all parts of your body.

Now, we shift our focus and awareness to our thoughts. Notice what is going on in your mind right now. What types of thoughts are you having? Is your mind occupied with racing thoughts? Or is your mind fairly inactive right now? Just note where your mind is. Notice if you are having trouble focusing today, or if you are completely relaxed and feeling at peace.

Lastly, we bring our awareness to our feelings today. What are you feeling right now? What emotion or emotions might you be experiencing? Emotions can change very easily, and we could be feeling multiple emotions at the same time, so just know that it is okay, whatever you are experiencing. Is something bothering you or frustrating you? Are you excited and eager about something? Are you feeling worried or anxious right now? Whatever it is, just sit with it for a moment and get curious about why you are feeling this way. You may be unsure of what you are feeling, and that is perfectly okay as well. There is no right or wrong here.

Now, bring your attention to taking five slow breaths in and out of your nose, and when you are ready, you may open your eyes.

Pregame Mindfulness Activities: For All Sports

***

Visualization One

Breathing Exercise:

Inhale for four seconds, hold for seven seconds, and exhale for eight seconds. Repeat this breathing sequence five times.

Positive Affirmations & Self-Compassion

Take a moment to close your eyes and settle into a comfortable position. Allow your body to relax and let go of tension, worries, or stress. Tell your body to relax and let go, making sure you are not holding on to any unwanted tension in your body. Every muscle should be soft, loosening, and lengthening. Use your breathing to allow the body to settle in for this visualization.

We are going to repeat some positive affirmations to ourselves right now. I want you to repeat these affirmations, with conviction, to yourself silently.

I am enough.
I know I have talent.
I know how to play this game well, and I will focus on that.

I can only do my best.

I will be successful during this game.

I am a great player.

I am in control of my emotions at all times.

I am NOT my performance.

I will be kind to myself during the game.

It's okay to make a mistake.

It's okay to have a bad day or performance.

I will let go of my fears.

I will play for myself and not compare myself to others.

I will look at everything as a learning experience for personal growth.

I will bounce back quickly when I have a setback.

I am ready for this; I am strong, I am confident.

I can do this.

I will succeed!

Now, bring your attention to three natural breaths, keeping your attention and focus on each inhale and each exhale. When you are ready, you may open your eyes.

Visualization Two

Breathing Exercise:

Let's take a moment to focus on our breath. Let's start out by taking three breaths, where we extend our exhale a little longer than our inhale, allowing our body to slow down.

Body Scan:

Let's take a moment to scan your body for any areas of stress and tension, starting with your feet, allowing your feet to soften and relax, moving up to your ankles, your calves, your knees, and your upper legs. Imagine softening and loosening all of these muscles. Then, moving around to the back of the legs, we are making sure they are relaxed. Now, focus on your hips, softening them and letting go of tension. Focus on your belly, allowing it to relax, and then move up to the chest, releasing tension. Bring the focus around to your back, allowing this area to let go completely, relaxing your shoulders, neck, face, and head. Now, take a moment to notice your body as a whole, allowing it to relax.

Visualization of my Best Game:

I want you to visualize your best game.

Remember back to a game that you played extremely well. Picture yourself there right now.

Remember the way the game went, in vivid detail.

Picture yourself and your teammates making specific plays that were executed perfectly.

Remember a specific play you made personally.

Remember exactly how you made that play and what led up to the play.

What were you thinking, what was going on? What did you hear? Imagine all the details of this play.

Now, think about the feelings you had while making that play.

Let those feelings grow inside of you now. Let the feelings of positivity, success, motivation, drive, happiness, excitement, and teamwork take over your mind.

Imagine going out today/tonight with that same great attitude and determination that you will play well, stay focused, and work well with your team.

Please take a deep breath, in through your nose and out through your nose. When you are ready, you may open your eyes.

Visualization Three

Breathing Exercise: Beach Ball Breath (Harper et al.,2017)

Begin by finding a comfortable seated position. Put your arms out in front of you with your fingers touching and imagine that you are holding a big beach ball. As you inhale, open your arms out to the sides, stretching out your chest, and lifting your chin. Then, as you exhale, bring your arms back together, as you round your back and bring your chin to your chest. Continue to do this at least five times.

Visualization: Paying Attention to the Mind, Body, and Breathing

Find a comfortable position and begin to settle in. Close your eyes or gaze downward. We are going to spend a few moments tuning into what is going on within ourselves at this moment.

It is important to remember that your body and your mind provide you with useful information if you listen to them. When you start becoming aware of this information, you can begin to help yourself by learning to calm down, get into your zone, and get out of your head. This can impact your timing, your ability, and your performance in a game in a positive way.

Let's take a moment to notice what is going on in your mind. Notice what thoughts are present right now, if any. Notice what feelings or emotions are present for you, if any.

Let's take a moment to notice how your body feels right now. Scan through your entire body, noticing what feels relaxed, what may hurt, if any area is sore, or if any area is loose. Notice any other sensations that are present in your body as well.

Let's take a moment to focus on your breathing. Notice how you are breathing right now. Are your breaths shallow or deep, slow or rapid, easy or difficult? Just notice how you are breathing in this moment.

Now let's focus on our intentions for this game.

Take a moment to think of what your personal intention is for tonight's or today's game. It could be something like, play hard, play smooth, stay in control, be grateful, stay positive, stay focused. Choose something you want to focus on for the game and repeat it three times to yourself right now.

Visualize what you want to happen tonight/today. Imagine yourself going out there tonight/today and playing your best game. See your moves; see your plays; see your speed and efficiency. Visualize it all right now with vivid detail. See the score. Watch your teammates and the fans, excited for this game.

Now, bring your attention to an inhalation and an exhalation.
I would like you to repeat these affirmations to yourself:
I am a great player.
I move efficiently and effectively.
I am motivated.
I am confident.
I am successful.
I am a winner!
When you are ready, you may slowly open your eyes.

Visualization Four

Breathing Exercise: Counting Breaths

Sit in a comfortable position and begin by bringing your attention and awareness to your breathing. Notice how you are breathing right now; shallow, deep, fast, slow. Just notice, no need to try to change anything at all. Now, I want you to begin to count your breaths. For example, as you inhale, count one, and as you exhale, count two. Continue to count this way until you reach ten. When you get to ten, you can restart from number one again. If you get lost in counting and find you are way over ten, that is completely fine. When you notice that you have lost track, bring yourself back to counting from one again. (Continue for about one minute). Now, notice how you feel. Do you feel more relaxed? Is your mind still very active? Remember, whatever is going on is fine the way it is.

Visualization: Building Self-Esteem

I want you to picture yourself at a time in your life when you were really happy. Be picky and remember a time that completely stands out to you. Take a moment to remember how you felt, remembering feeling joy, happiness, and excitement. Picture yourself at that time, feeling so good. It might even bring a smile to your face when you reminisce about this time. Can you notice any feelings in your body when you are thinking of this time when you felt great? Perhaps you might notice a feeling of lightness, warmth, openness, or comfort. Take a moment to soak up those wonderful feelings.

Now, as you are feeling great, I want you to offer yourself some kind words for tonight's/today's game.

Say these affirmations to yourself now:

I am a worthwhile person.
I am unique, and I appreciate my uniqueness.
I feel good about myself.
It is okay to like myself.

I deserve to be happy.

I am perfectly alright, just the way I am.

I do not need to compare myself to others.

I have many good qualities.

I am a great player.

I have so much talent and ability.

I am a hard worker.

I will put forth my greatest effort today/tonight.

I will stay positive and focused on playing well.

I will use my self-confidence and these positive affirmations in tonight's/today's game.

Bring your attention back to an inhalation and an exhalation.

When you are ready, you can open your eyes.

Visualization Five

Breathing Exercise:

Get into a comfortable position, seated in your chair or lying on the floor. Let's bring your focus to your breath, and as you breathe in, I want you to imagine breathing in light and success. As you breathe out, I want you to visualize darkness and negativity leaving your body. You are allowing light and success into the body and getting rid of any negativity. Continue to breathe like this for a few breaths.

Visualization: Focusing and Noticing

Now, begin by relaxing your muscles and allowing everything to soften and release. Tell your body to relax and let go. Notice any areas of tension, tightness, or discomfort, and pay particular attention to those areas, giving them special care to relax. Notice your entire body resting on the surface you are on now. Can you feel your body as a whole? Can you allow your body to soften and sink into the surface a little deeper? Hopefully, now your body is relaxed, so we can move on to the mind.

Notice what thoughts are going through your head right now. Are they positive? Negative? Neutral? For a moment, let's pretend that each thought you have, has floated into the sky and away on a cloud. As each thought pops into your head, just visualize it floating on a cloud in the sky, moving far away. It is important to allow your mind to slow down so that you can stay grounded and focused on your performance.

Let's begin by trying to focus our attention on one thing at a time. Allow yourself to bring your focus to your feet. What sensations or feelings do you notice in your feet? Do you notice warmth or coolness; tingling or pulsing; lightness or heaviness?

Now, bring your attention to one full breath in, and one full breath out.

Bring your awareness to your hands. Maybe you notice your hands touching or your hands resting in your lap. Can you feel any sensations in your hands? Can you feel your hands?

Now, bring your attention to your breathing. As you inhale, follow your inhale, and as you exhale, follow your exhale.

Next, bring your attention to your shoulders. Notice if you can sense tightness, heaviness, lightness, or looseness in your shoulders. If you do sense tightness, allow your shoulders to soften and move away from your ears.

Bring your attention to a full breath in and a full breath out. Allow your attention to rest with the breath for a moment. Feel how natural and easy your breathing is right now.

Now, bring your attention to where your body is touching the surface you are on right now. Can you notice your body's weight sinking down into the chair or floor?

Can you notice your feet? Can you feel any sensations, pulsing, feelings of warmth or coolness, tingling, itching, or perhaps nothing in your feet?

Can you bring your attention to a time when you were successful? This can be any time that pops into your head, when you hear the words "success", "victory", or "triumph". Think about this time in your life and bring it to the forefront of your mind. Feel your success, feel your victory, feel your triumph, and feel your enthusiasm. Allow these feelings to continue to expand and spread all over your being.

I want you to take these same feelings with you for today's/ tonight's game and remember that you choose how you want to feel.

Take a deep breath in through your nose and out through your nose. Open your eyes.

Visualization Six

Internal Motivation:

Let's begin by finding a comfortable seated position, with the spine elongated and straight, but soft. Let your shoulders release and drop away from your ears and allow your body to soften. Starting from the top of your head, allow each body part I mention to soften, release, and let go; head, face, neck, shoulders, chest, back, and hips. Allow those areas to melt into relaxation and release all tension. Now, move to your upper arms, lower arms, and hands, softening these muscles. Now, work your way to the lower body, relaxing your thighs, back of the legs, calves, shins, and feet. From your head to your toes, every part of your body should be completely relaxed.

Let's focus now on getting into your zone today. Getting into your zone means this is the time when you do your best, you perform well, you achieve high, and you are at the top of your game. You do not allow distractions to get in the way of your goal, which is to play your best. Take a moment to visualize what being in your zone looks and feels like. To do this, it might be helpful to visualize how you want to play. See yourself executing plays with ease, speed, and efficiency. Imagine in your mind that you are playing your best game, performing at your best, and feeling your best.

Visualize yourself playing a mistake-free game. What does that look and feel like? Your offense is strong, confident, and precise. Your defense is also strong, unstoppable, and unbreakable. Imagine what perfect offense and defense looks like in this game. Picture some of the plays you have discussed with your coach and see you and your teammates executing those plays with accuracy.

Please repeat these affirmations to yourself for some positive encouragement for the game:

I am ready for this game.

I am ready to play my best.

I am ready to be efficient, accurate, and execute all plays well.

I am ready to be strong, confident, and unstoppable.

I am ready to win!

Take a deep breath, in through your nose and out through your nose.

When you are ready, you may open your eyes.

BASKETBALL VISUALIZATIONS

***

Visualization One

Breathing Exercise:

As we breathe today, I want you to say to yourself, "**I am confident**" each time you inhale, and say to yourself, "**I am strong**" as you exhale. Continue to do this a few times, each time repeating, I am confident on the inhale, and I am strong on the exhale. Allow yourself to settle in and get ready for this visualization.

Imagining A Positive Game:

Imagine walking into the gym, feeling confident, strong, and ready to perform well. See yourself walking with pep in your step, standing tall and proud, and feeling ready to take on this team.

Imagine yourself starting your warm-up.

See your warm-up going exactly the way you want it to. Feel the positive energy, the excitement, and the intense focus you have on getting and staying in your zone.

See yourself at the top of the key, making ten free throws. As you shoot, I want you to feel the ball roll off your fingers, see the ball traveling through the air with perfect backspin, see your hands out in front of you with the perfect follow-through, see your hands in front of you, holding your follow-through as you hear and see the ball swish through the net each and every time.

Now, let's visualize during the game.

What will you say to yourself during the game to keep you motivated and focused?

Examples could be, stay focused, you got this, you know what you are doing, two points every time you shoot, focus, follow-through, stay calm.

Pick one that works for you and say that affirmation to yourself now.

Take a moment to visualize what you want to happen tonight/today, and how you want to play and perform.

Take a deep breath, in through your nose and out through your nose. When you are ready, you may open your eyes.

Visualization Two

Breathing: Elephant Breath (Guber et al. 2005)

Standing tall, take a big deep breath in, as you raise your arms above you, and as you exhale, you let your arms swing between your legs like an elephant's trunk, letting the head and neck go. Roll up like a rag doll. Do this at least five times.

Visualize Your Game:

Imagine that your body is in tip-top condition today.

You feel great!

You are sending positive energy to all of your muscles and body parts.

Imagine and feel that everything is flowing, and you are ready physically for this game.

Imagine yourself entering the gym today and starting your warm-up.

Imagine your routine and what you will say to yourself to pump yourself up with positivity.

Imagine your warm-up going very well.

Now, imagine being on the court; you are aware of the other people around you, and the people in the crowd. You can hear noises in the gym, but none of this matters to you because you are giving your attention to shooting, practicing, and playing.

Imagine all of your shots going in, with a swoosh.

Feel your perfect form and flow.

You are in your zone, not letting distractions break your focus.

It feels natural and easy to make these shots.

Imagine making your three-pointers with ease and focus.

Imagine standing at the top of the key, you begin to shoot, taking one shot after the other, each one going in smoothly.

You are now warmed up and ready to play at the top of your game.

You will let mistakes go easily and move on quickly.

You will let nothing stand in your way of playing great.

You will stay focused.

You will play the game you love to play.

Bring your attention to your breath. Take three slow deep breaths, in through your nose and out through your nose. When you are ready, you may open your eyes.

Visualization Three

Breathing Exercise: Heart and Belly Breathing

Place one hand on your heart and the other on your belly. Continue to breathe normally and naturally as you focus your attention on the pace of your breathing. You should notice that your breathing slows down when your hands are in this position. As you breathe, send kind wishes to yourself. You can say to yourself:

I am strong.
I am confident.
I am proud of who I am.
I am successful.

I am a winner!

After you repeat these affirmations to yourself, you may allow your hands to fall to your sides or rest in your lap.

We will begin the visualization now.

Recalling a Time:

I want you to remember when and why you wanted to play ball.

Bring yourself back to the time when you were first interested in the game. See where you were, who you were with, and how you felt, playing this game.

Remember what you love about this game. Let those memories come to you and notice the positive feelings it brings up.

Now, imagine being on the court right now. I want you to take three long, slow deep breaths, in through the nose and out through the mouth. Stay in the moment with each breath you take.

You are ready to play tonight/today! You will use your breathing to help relax and calm yourself down if you feel you are getting too emotional or upset. You will turn your focus inward.

Now, take a moment to see yourself making shots. Imagine making a few lay-ups and imagine making some three pointers. Feel your body in alignment as you make each shot. Feel the ball roll off your fingertips, and see the perfect backspin on each shot. What will you say to yourself before you make each shot that will help motivate you tonight? You want to think of something quick and easy to say, for instance; two points; each shot counts; I've got this; focus; smooth. Choose a phrase or word that works for you, and I want you to picture yourself setting up for a shot and saying this before each shot.

Now, take a moment to focus on free throws. Imagine yourself standing at the free-throw line. Your feet are planted on the gym floor, and your body is in alignment. You take your shot, and it goes in. Again, what will you say to yourself each time you have to make a free throw? Practice what you will say to yourself now.

Lastly, visualize a few key plays that you have discussed with your coach, and see yourself and your teammates acting out perfectly each play. Everyone is positioned correctly and working together, exactly how you planned. You execute each play with perfection and ease.

You are ready to play and ready to win. You are ready to show everyone what you are made of and how skilled your team is!

Remember to breathe. Stop and take five breaths if you need to at any point during the game.

Visualization Four

Breathing Exercise: Calming Your Breath

Let's start by taking a deep, slow breath in through your nose, and then release your breath through your nose or mouth. Take one more slow, deep breath. Now, continue breathing naturally and normally. Breathing in calm and peace, breathing out stress and tension.

The Perfect Game:

Let go of the tension in each part of your body;

Soften your face, eyes, neck;

Drop your shoulders;

Feel your arms getting heavy and relaxed.

Move to your lower body;

Relaxing every muscle in your upper legs, lower legs, and feet.

As you relax, you can begin visualizing yourself playing basketball, the sport that you love.

You are warming up on the court, feeling confident and excited for this game. You can see your teammates around you, who are also pumped up and ready to play.

You are focused and have a positive mindset for this game.

You know you will perform to the best of your ability.

You are bringing your A game.

You came to be successful!

Now, picture yourself holding the ball in your hands. Imagine dribbling quickly and moving around the court with grace and ease. You feel in control, and you will not let anyone stand in your way. Imagine yourself dribbling strong and smooth as you jog down the court. Imagine what you will do when a defender comes your way. See yourself easily dribbling around them. You feel confident in handling and moving the ball around the court. You are staying in each moment, focusing on one play and one move at a time. Imagine passing the ball to your teammate with precision and accuracy. You and your teammates are making smart plays. You feel mentally and physically in tip top shape for this game. Now, imagine yourself taking a lay-up. Your shot is smooth, and you score! Imagine yourself running down the court with fast feet and great timing. Everything is falling into place, and the game is going the way you want it to. You are shooting with accuracy, you are moving with speed and ease, you are playing with determination and focus.

Now, bring your attention back to your breathing. Notice how you feel now as opposed to the beginning of the visualization. When you are ready, you may open your eyes.

LACROSSE VISUALIZATIONS

---✦---

Visualization One

Breathing Exercise:

As you breathe today, I want you to say to yourself, **"I am confident"** each time you inhale, and say to yourself, **"I am strong"** as you exhale. Continue to do this a few times, each time repeating, I am confident on the inhale, and I am strong on the exhale. Allow yourself to settle in and get ready for this visualization.

Imagining a Positive Game:

Imagine walking onto the field, feeling confident, strong, and ready to perform well. See yourself walking with pep in your step, standing tall and proud, and feeling ready to take on this team.

Imagine yourself starting your warm-up.

See your warm-up and everything going the way you want it to. Feel the positive energy, the excitement, and the intense focus you have on getting and staying in your zone.

What will you say to yourself when you are warming up? I am in control; I can do this; I will be a success; I am a great player?

Pick one of these positive affirmations, and repeat the positive affirmation to yourself right now, three times in silence.

Now, let's begin to visualize in detail how you are executing your practice. See yourself practicing and making five goals in a row. As you set up for your shot on goal, I want you to feel your hands handling the stick, cradling back and forth with perfect speed and technique; feel your body easily moving with quick, fast, agile movements; see the ball traveling through the air; hitting the back of the net, and scoring a goal.

Take a moment to truly visualize all of this and feel it.

Now, we will visualize what will happen during the game.

What will you say to yourself during the game to keep you motivated and focused?

Examples could be, stay focused, you got this, you know what you are doing, focus, be fast and efficient, stay calm.

Pick one that works for you and say that affirmation to yourself now.

Take a moment to visualize what you want to happen today and how you want to play and perform. Visualize yourself taking your position on the field and owning that position. See yourself play this position with precision.

Bring your attention to the flow of your breathing as you follow each inhalation and each exhalation fully. Each breath is calming and relaxing you, getting you ready for the game.

When you are ready, you can open your eyes.

Visualization Two

Breathing: Elephant Breath

Standing tall, take a big deep breath in, as you raise your arms above you, and as you exhale, you let your arms swing between your legs like an elephant's trunk, letting the head and neck go. Roll up like a rag doll. Do this at least five times.

Visualize Your Game:

Imagine that your body is in tip-top condition today.

You feel great!

You are sending positive energy to all of your muscles and body parts.

Imagine and feel that everything is flowing, and you are ready physically for this game.

Imagine yourself entering the field today and starting your warm-up.

Imagine your routine and what you will say to yourself to pump yourself up with positivity.

Imagine your warm-up going very well.

Now, imagine being on the field, and you are aware of the other people around you, and the people in the crowd. You can hear noises on the field, but none of this matters to you because you are giving your attention to shooting, practicing, and playing.

Imagine all of your shots going in the goal, imagine your footwork and agility are on point.

Feel your perfect form and flow.

You are in your zone, not letting distractions break your focus.

It feels natural and easy to make these goals.

Imagine making your goals with ease and focus. Visualize all of your passes to your teammates are precise and accurate.

You are now warmed up and ready to play at the top of your game!

You will let mistakes go easily and move on quickly.

You will let nothing stand in your way of playing great.

You will stay focused.

You will play the game you love to play!

When you are ready, you may open your eyes.

Visualization Three

Breathing: Heart and Belly Breathing

Place one hand on your heart and the other on your belly. Continue to breathe normally and naturally as you focus your attention on the pace of your breathing. You should notice that your breathing slows down when your hands are in this position. As you breathe, send kind wishes to yourself. You can say to yourself:

I am strong.
I am confident.
I am proud of who I am.
I am successful.
I am a winner!

After you repeat these affirmations to yourself, you may allow your hands to fall to your sides or rest in your lap.

We will begin the visualization now.

Recalling a Time:

Let's recall the very first time you played lacrosse. Can you remember this time? Can you picture the details? Where were you? Who were you with? What was going on around you? Let's take a moment to recall this special time that you fell in the love with this game and decided that you wanted to play lacrosse competitively. Soak in the memory and allow it to fill your mind's eye. Let the memory fill you up with joy, energy, positivity, and happiness.

Allow those positive feelings and feelings of determination, motivation, dedication, and drive to fill you up and spread to every part of your being. Soak up all of those wonderful feelings of the time when you connected with the game. Try to take those wonderful feelings with you in today's game, and have fun playing this game.

Now, imagine being on the field right now. I want you to take three long, slow deep breaths in through the nose and out through the mouth. Stay in the moment with each breath you take.

You are ready to play today. You will use your breathing to help relax and calm yourself down if you feel you are getting too emotional or upset. You will turn your focus inward and stay in your zone.

Now, take a moment to see yourself making successful passes. Imagine making some smooth, quick, confident passes to your teammates. Feel your body in alignment as you make each pass. Feel your hands, cradling the stick, and see your teammates in perfect position. What will you say to yourself before you make each pass and play that will help motivate you today? You want to think of something quick and easy to say, for instance; every pass counts; I've got this; focus; smooth; be quick. Choose a phrase or word that works for you, and I want you to picture yourself setting up for a pass, taking a shot on goal, or executing a play, and saying this before each time.

Now, take a moment to focus on your position on the field and your footwork. Imagine yourself standing on the field in your ready position. Your body is in alignment, your hand position is accurate, and you wait for the signal to start. Imagine your movement, your speed, and the feel of your body as you prepare to begin the game. Take a moment to visualize this now.

Lastly, visualize a few key plays that you have discussed with your coach and see yourself and your teammates acting out perfectly each play. Everyone is positioned correctly and working together, exactly the way you planned. You execute each play with perfection and ease.

You are ready to play and ready to win. You are ready to show everyone what you are made of and how skilled your team is!

Remember to breathe. Stop and take five breaths if you need to at any point during the game.

Visualization Four

Breathing Exercise:

Let's start out by bringing your attention to your breath. Let's see if you can focus on each inhale and each exhale. Can you notice where you are feeling your breath the most today? Do you feel the air moving in and out of your nostrils, or can you feel your chest rise and fall as you breathe, or maybe you notice your belly rising and falling as you breathe? Pick one of these three areas where you most naturally and easily feel your breath. Know that your breathing is always here for you as your anchor, grounding and stabilizing you when you need it.

Body Scan:

Next, allow your body to relax and soften. Starting at the top of your head, relax each body part as you work your way down your body. Allow the face to soften, the neck to relax, the shoulders to drop, the chest to release, and the arms and hands to relax. Move around to your back and allow this area to completely let go of tension; the hips begin to soften; the legs begin to release and elongate, and the feet and toes begin to let go. Your entire body should be completely relaxed and ready to focus on our visualization for today.

Set the Scene:

I want you to create a picture in your mind of the lacrosse field you play on every day. Picture the details of this field, and imagine you are standing on the field admiring the scenery. Look around at the bleachers, the press box, the score board, and then the field itself. This is the game that you love to play. You feel confident, important, and proud when you play this game. Take a moment to allow those great feelings, and the feelings of excitement to spread throughout your whole body.

Now, imagine you are getting ready to enter the field with your teammates. You are pumped up, excited, eager, full of energy and positivity. You are ready to play this game and to play it well. Feel what it feels like, standing there with your team getting ready to enter the field. What do you notice? What can you hear? What can you see, people in the bleachers, coaches, players, friends? Soak it all in.

Now, you are ready to make your entrance. You run onto the field and start your warm-up. Visualize your warm-up going smoothly and exactly the way you want it to. Take a moment to imagine feeling strong, fast, efficient, pumped up, and ready to play your best.

You know this game, your body knows this game, and your heart knows this game. You love to play, and you love to play well. Feel yourself getting into your zone where you are unstoppable, unbeatable, and unbreakable. Feel confident in your ability as a player, feel strong in your presence, feel grounded in your body and mind.

This is your moment to shine; this is your game to claim; this is your time to achieve success. Feel it, believe it, and allow it!

Bring your focus to your breathing. Notice the air coming into the nostrils and the air leaving the nostrils. Take one big deep breath in and release. When you are ready, you may open your eyes.

FOOTBALL VISUALIZATIONS

Visualization One

Breathing Exercise:

Let's start out by bringing your attention to your breath. Let's see if you can focus on each inhale and each exhale. Can you notice where you are feeling your breath the most today? Do you feel the air moving in and out of your nostrils, or can you feel your chest rise and fall as you breathe, or maybe you notice your belly rising and falling as you breathe? Pick one of these three areas where you most naturally and easily feel your breath. Know that your breathing is always here for you as your anchor, grounding and stabilizing you when you need it.

Body Scan:

Next, allow your body to relax and soften. Starting at the top of your head, relax each body part as you work your way down your body. Allow the face to soften, the neck to relax, the shoulders to drop, the chest to release, and the arms and hands to relax. Move around to your back and allow this area to completely let go of tension; the hips begin to soften; the legs begin to release and elongate, and the feet and toes begin to let go. Your entire body should be completely relaxed and ready to focus on our visualization for today.

Set the Scene:

I want you to create a picture in your mind of the football field you play on every day. Picture the details of this field, and imagine you are standing on the field admiring the scenery. Look around at the bleachers, the press box, the track, and then the field itself. This is the game that you love to play. You feel confident, important, and proud when you play this game. Take a moment to allow those great feelings, and the feelings of excitement to spread throughout your whole body.

Now, imagine you are getting ready to enter the field with your teammates. You are pumped up, excited, eager, full of energy and positivity. You are ready to play this game and to play it well. Feel what it feels like, standing there with your team getting ready to enter the field. What do you notice? What can you hear? Perhaps you can hear the crowd, cheerleaders, music playing, people talking. What can you see, people in the bleachers, coaches, players, friends? Soak it all in.

Now, you are ready to make your entrance. You run onto the field and start your warm-up. Visualize your warm-up going smoothly and exactly the way you want it to. Take a moment to imagine feeling strong, fast, efficient, pumped up, and ready to play your best.

You know this game, your body knows this game, and your heart knows this game. You love to play, and you love to play well. Feel yourself getting into your zone where you are unstoppable, unbeatable, and unbreakable. Feel confident in your ability as a player, feel strong in your presence, feel grounded in your body and mind.

This is your moment to shine; this is your game to claim; this is your time to achieve success. Feel it, believe it, and allow it!

Bring your focus to your breathing. Notice the air coming into the nostrils and the air leaving the nostrils. Take one big deep breath in and release. When you are ready, you may open your eyes.

Visualization Two

Beach Ball Breathing:

Begin by finding a comfortable, seated position. Put your arms in front of you with your hands touching and imagine that you are holding a big beach ball. As you inhale, open your arms out to the sides, opening your chest, and lifting your chin. As you exhale, bring your arms back together as you round your back and bring your chin to your chest. Continue to do this at least five times.

Recalling A Time:

Let's recall the very first time you played football. Can you remember this time? Can you picture the details? Where were you? Who were you with? What was going on around you? Let's take a moment to recall this special time when you fell in love with this game and decided that you wanted to play football competitively. Soak in the memory and allow it to fill your mind's eye. Let the memory fill you up with joy, energy, positivity, and happiness.

Allow those positive feelings and feelings of determination, motivation, dedication, and drive to fill you up and spread to every part of your being. Soak up all of those wonderful feelings, as you remember the time when you connected with the game. Now, try to take those wonderful feelings with you in today's game, and have fun playing this game.

Now, picture yourself in amazing physical shape. Feel and know that your body is strong, fast, agile, balanced, and full of energy. Your mind is in a positive state for today's/ tonight's game. You are pumped up and psyched for this game. You cannot wait to go out there today and play hard and play smart.

Allow yourself to truly visualize and feel that you are physically and mentally operating at peak levels. You are in your zone of perfect flow; nothing can break this zone.

Take a moment to visualize yourself playing your position today to the very best of your ability. Feel your strength, motivation, and determination for the game. Picture in your mind being on the field, facing your opponent with confidence, knowing that you are fully capable and ready for this game.

Now, bring the focus back to your body, making sure to release any tension. Take a deep breath, in through your nose and out through your nose. When you are ready, you may open your eyes.

Visualization Three

Breathing Exercise:

As you breathe today, I want you to say to yourself, **"I am confident"** each time you inhale, and say to yourself, **"I am strong"** as you exhale. Continue to do this a few times, each time repeating, I am confident on the inhale, and I am strong on the exhale. Allow yourself to settle in and get ready for this visualization.

Imagining A Positive Game:

Imagine walking onto the field, feeling confident, strong, and ready to perform well. See yourself walking with pep in your step, standing tall and proud, and feeling ready to take on this team. Hear the cheering from the crowd, the music playing, and all the excitement in the air.

Imagine yourself starting your warm-up.

What will you say to yourself when you are warming up? I am in control; I can do this, I will be a success, I am a great player?

Pick one phrase you feel will work for you during this game today/tonight that will help you stay on track. When you have this phrase, repeat this positive affirmation to yourself silently right now three times.

Now, see yourself executing your warm-up and everything going the way you want it to. Feel the positive energy, the excitement, and the intense focus you have on getting and staying in your zone.

See yourself practicing on the field, making efficient passes, making effortless catches, defending with strength and confidence, running with great speed, kicking field goals with accuracy. Imagine and visualize all of the aspects of this game that you are responsible for on the field, playing your position. Your warm-up is successful and precise.

Now, let's focus on what will happen during the game.

What will you say to yourself during the game to keep you motivated and focused?

Examples could be; stay focused, you got this, you know what you are doing, be fast and efficient, stay calm.

Pick one that works for you and repeat this affirmation to yourself silently three times.

Now, I want you to feel yourself in your position right now on the field. Feel the adrenaline pumping, feel your excitement and positive energy swirling around, feel your body strong and able, and ready for this game.

Take a moment to visualize what you want to happen today/tonight and how you want to play and perform. Then, take a deep breath, in through your nose and out through your nose. You are ready to play football!

Visualization Four

Breathing: Elephant Breath

Standing tall, take a big deep breath in, as you raise your arms above you, and as you exhale, you let your arms swing between your legs like an elephant's trunk, letting the head and neck go. Roll up like a rag doll. Do this at least five times.

Visualize Your Game:

Imagine that your body is in tip-top condition today.

You feel great!

You are sending positive energy to all of your muscles and body parts.

Imagine and feel that everything is flowing, and you are ready physically for this game.

Imagine yourself entering the field today and starting your warm-up.

Imagine your routine and what you will say to yourself to pump yourself up with positivity.

Imagine your warm-up going very well.

Now, imagine being on the field, and you are aware of the other people around you, and the people in the crowd. You can hear noises on the field, but none of this matters to you because you are focusing your attention on throwing, catching, and playing.

Imagine all of your passes are being perfectly executed.

Imagine your movement on the field is on point. Your defense is strong and your offense is fast.

Feel your perfect form and flow while making successful catches and throws.

You are in your zone, not letting distraction break your focus.

It feels natural and easy to make these plays.

Imagine executing practice plays with ease, focus, and strength.

You are now warmed up and ready to play at the top of your game.

You will let mistakes go easily and move on quickly.

You will let nothing stand in your way of playing great.

You will stay focused.

You will play the game you love to play!

When you are ready, you may open your eyes.

BASEBALL VISUALIZATIONS

✳

Visualization One

Breathing Exercise:

As we breathe today, I want you to say to yourself, "**I am confident**" each time you inhale, and say to yourself, "**I am strong**", as you exhale. Continue to do this a few times, each time repeating, I am confident on the inhale, and I am strong on the exhale. Allow yourself to settle in and get ready for this visualization.

Imagining A Positive Game:

Imagine walking onto the field, feeling confident, strong, and ready to perform well. See yourself walking with pep in your step, standing tall and proud, and feeling ready to take on this team.

Imagine yourself starting your warm-up.

What will you say to yourself when you are warming up? I am in control; I can do this; I will be a success; I am a great player? Choose an affirmation that feels right for you, and repeat this positive affirmation silently to yourself right now.

See yourself warming-up and everything going the way you want it to. Feel the positive energy, the excitement, and the intense focus you have on getting and staying in your zone.

See yourself throwing and catching with a teammate. The skills are natural and easy for you. As you practice hitting, I want you to feel your grip on the bat, feel your body in your set up position. You are in perfect alignment. See the pitcher release the ball, see yourself following the ball as it gets closer to you. Feel yourself getting ready for your swing, and then feel yourself make contact with the ball and follow through with all of your strength. See your direct contact with the ball and the ball flying long and high into the field. Continue to visualize hitting with accuracy, strength, and confidence. You are making great hits each time you practice.

Now, let's begin to visualize what will happen during the game.

What will you say to yourself during the game to keep you motivated and focused?

Examples could be; stay focused, you got this, you know what you are doing, keep your eye on the ball, stay calm. Pick one that works for you and repeat that affirmation to yourself now.

Take a moment to visualize what you want to happen today/tonight and how you want to play and perform. Then take a deep breath, in through your nose and out through your nose. You are ready to play baseball!

Visualization Two

Breathing: Heart and Belly Breathing

Place one hand on your heart and the other on your belly. Continue to breathe normally and naturally as you focus your attention on the pace of your breathing. You should notice that your breathing slows down when your hands are in this position. As you breathe, send kind wishes to yourself. You can say to yourself:

I am strong.
I am confident.
I am proud of who I am.
I am successful.
I am a winner!

After you repeat these affirmations to yourself, you may allow your hands to fall to your sides or rest in your lap.

We will begin the visualization now.

Recalling a Time:

I want you to remember when and why you wanted to play baseball. Can you remember this time? Can you picture the details? Where were you? Who were you with? What was going on around you? Let's take a moment to recall this special time when you fell in love with this game and decided that you wanted to play baseball competitively. Soak in the memory and allow it to fill your mind's eye. Let the memory fill you up with joy, energy, positivity, and happiness.

Allow those positive feelings, and feelings of determination, motivation, dedication, and drive to fill you up and spread to every part of your being. Soak up all of those wonderful feelings of the time when you connected with this game. Now, try to take those wonderful feelings with you into today's game, and have fun playing this game.

Now, imagine being on the field right now. I want you to take three long, slow deep breaths, in through the nose and out through the mouth. Stay in the moment with each breath you take.

You are ready to play today/tonight. You will use your breathing to help relax and calm yourself down if you feel you are getting too emotional or upset. You will turn your focus inward and stay in your zone.

Now, take a moment to see yourself up at-bat. Imagine making some great hits and imagine making some beautiful catches. Feel your body in alignment as you take each hit. See the ball as it approaches your glove, and you make the perfect catch. Visualize making some great plays. See yourself and your teammates working together in the field, making outs.

What will you say to yourself before you are up at bat that will help motivate you today/tonight? You want to think of something quick and easy to say, for instance, every hit counts; I've got this; focus; smooth; concentrate. Choose a phrase or word that works for you, and I want you to picture yourself up at bat, pitching, catching, or taking a field position and saying this before each play.

Now, take a moment to focus on outfield plays. Imagine yourself standing in your position on the field. Take a look at your teammates and notice where each one is located. You are completely aware of your surroundings and focused on the next play. Imagine yourself in your ready position as the opponent is up at-bat. See the opponent make a hit, follow the ball, and visualize yourself and your teammates making the catch and getting the out.

Lastly, visualize a few key plays that you have discussed with your coach, and see yourself and your teammates acting out perfectly each play. Everyone is positioned correctly and working together, exactly the way you planned. You execute each play with perfection and ease.

You are ready to play and ready to win. You are ready to show everyone what you are made of and how skilled your team is!

Remember to breathe. Stop and take five breaths if you need to at any point during the game.

Visualization Three

Breathing: Elephant Breath

Standing tall, take a big deep breath in, as you raise your arms above you, and as you exhale, you let your arms swing between your legs like an elephant's trunk, letting the head and neck go. Roll up like a rag doll. Do this at least five times.

Visualize Your Game:

Imagine that your body is in tip-top condition today.

You feel great!

You are sending positive energy to all of your muscles and body parts.

Imagine and feel that everything is flowing, and you are ready physically for this game.

Imagine yourself entering the field today and starting your warm-up.

Imagine your routine and what you will say to yourself to pump yourself up with positivity.

Imagine your warm-up going very well.

Now, imagine being on the field, and you are aware of the other people around you, and the people in the crowd. You can hear noises on the field, but none of this matters to you because you are focusing your attention on hitting, catching, and playing.

Imagine all of your swings being perfectly executed.
Imagine your movement on the field, going in for a catch is on point.
Feel your perfect form and flow while making successful catches and throws.
You are in your zone, not letting distraction break your focus.
It feels natural and easy to make these plays.
Imagine stepping up at batt with ease, focus, and strength.
You are now warmed up and ready to play at the top of your game.
You will let mistakes go easily and move on quickly.

You will let nothing stand in your way of playing great.

You will stay focused.

You will play the game you love to play!

When you are ready, you may open your eyes.

Visualization Four

Breathing Exercise:

Let's start out by bringing your attention to your breath. Let's see if you can focus on each inhale and each exhale. Can you notice where you are feeling your breath the most today? Do you feel the air moving in and out of your nostrils, or can you feel your chest rise and fall as you breathe, or maybe you notice your belly rising and falling as you breathe? Pick one of these three areas where you most naturally and easily feel your breath. Know that your breathing is always here for you as your anchor, grounding and stabilizing you when you need it.

Body Scan:

Next, allow your body to relax and soften. Starting at the top of your head, relax each body part as you work your way down your body. Allow the face to soften, the neck to relax, the shoulders to drop, the chest to release, and the arms and hands to relax. Move around to your back and allow this area to completely let go of tension; the hips begin to soften; the legs begin to release and elongate, and the feet and toes begin to let go. Your entire body should be completely relaxed and ready to focus on our visualization for today.

Set the Scene:

I want you to create a picture in your mind of the baseball field you play on every day. Picture the details of this field, and imagine you are standing on the field admiring the scenery. Look around at the bleachers, the dug-out, the score board, and then the field itself. This is the game that you love to play. You feel confident, important, and proud when you play this game. Take a moment to allow those great feelings, and the feelings of excitement to spread throughout your whole body.

Now, imagine you are getting ready to enter the field with your teammates. You are pumped up, excited, eager, full of energy and positivity. You are ready to play this game and to play it well. Feel what it feels like, standing there with your team getting ready to enter the field. What do you notice? What can you hear? What can you see, people in the bleachers, coaches, players, friends? Soak it all in.

Now, you are ready to make your entrance. You run onto the field and start your warm-up. Visualize your warm-up going smoothly and exactly the way you want it to. Take a moment to imagine feeling strong, fast, efficient, pumped up, and ready to play your best.

You know this game, your body knows this game, and your heart knows this game. You love to play, and you love to play well. Feel yourself getting into your zone where you are unstoppable, unbeatable, and unbreakable. Feel confident in your ability as a player, feel strong in your presence, feel grounded in your body and mind.

This is your moment to shine; this is your game to claim; this is your time to achieve success. Feel it, believe it, and allow it!

Bring your focus to your breathing. Notice the air coming into the nostrils and the air leaving the nostrils. Take one big deep breath in and release. When you are ready, you may open your eyes.

VOLLEYBALL VISUALIZATIONS

Visualization One

Breathing:

As we breathe today, I want you to say to yourself, "**I am confident**" each time you inhale and say to yourself, "**I am strong**" as you exhale. Continue to do this a few times, each time repeating I am confident on the inhale, and I am strong on the exhale. Allow yourself to settle in and get ready for this visualization.

Imagine A Positive Game:

Imagine walking into the gym, feeling confident, strong, and ready to perform well. See yourself walking with pep in your step, standing tall and proud, and feeling ready to take on this team.

Imagine yourself starting your warm-up.

What will you say to yourself when you are warming up? I am in control; I can do this; I will be a success; I am a great player? Pick one of these phrases that work for you and repeat the statement to yourself right now.

See yourself executing your warm-up and everything going the way you want it to. Feel the positive energy, the excitement, and the intense focus you have on getting and staying in your zone.

See yourself on the court, practicing with your team. Feel your perfect body alignment, see the ball coming toward you, feel your body setting up for a bump or set, feel how grounded and stable you are, feel yourself make contact with the ball with perfect form, see the ball landing exactly where you intended it to land. Visualize you and your teammates working together with perfect flow, positions, and movement on the court to successfully bump, set, spike. Imagine practicing a few sequences of bump, set, spike with your teammates. Feel how smooth, focused, and in a rhythm you are. You are in your zone.

Now, let's focus on what will happen during the game.

What will you say to yourself during the game to keep yourself motivated and focused?

Examples could be; stay focused, you got this, you know what you are doing, breathe, stay calm.

Pick one that works for you and repeat this affirmation silently to yourself now.

Take a moment to visualize what you want to happen today/tonight and how you want to play and perform. Visualize each play being executed with perfection. Imagine getting ready to serve; you are in your ready position; hands on the ball; you toss the ball into the air, following it with your eyes; you extend your arm, and smack the ball with the heel of your hand, as it travels over the net at high speed. The ball drops to the ground on your opponent's side. Your point! You are ready for this game!

Now, bring your attention back to your breathing and follow each inhale and exhale fully. When you are ready, you may open your eyes.

Visualization Two

Breathing: Heart and Belly Breathing

Place one hand on your heart and the other on your belly. Continue to breathe normally and naturally as you focus your attention on the pace of your breathing. You should notice that your breathing slows down when your hands are in this position. As you breathe, send kind wishes to yourself. You can say to yourself:

I am strong.
I am confident.
I am proud of who I am.
I am successful.
I am a winner!

After you repeat these affirmations to yourself, you may allow your hands to fall to your sides or rest in your lap.

We will begin the visualization now.

Recalling a Time:

I want you to remember when and why you wanted to play volleyball. Can you remember this time? Can you picture the details? Where were you? Who were you with? What was going on around you? Let's take a moment to recall this special time when you fell in love with this game and decided that you wanted to play volleyball competitively. Soak in the memory and allow it to fill your mind's eye. Let the memory fill you up with joy, energy, positivity, and happiness.

Allow those positive feelings and feelings of determination, motivation, dedication, and drive to fill you up and spread to every part of your being. Soak up all of those wonderful feelings of the time when you first connected with the game. Now, try to take those wonderful feelings with you in today's game, and have fun playing this game.

Imagine being on the court right now. I want you to take three long, slow deep breaths, in through the nose and out through the mouth. Stay in the moment with each breath you take.

You are ready to play today/tonight! You will use your breathing to help relax and calm yourself down if you feel you are getting too emotional or upset. You will turn your focus inward to stay in your zone.

Now, take a moment to see yourself making passes. Imagine yourself setting up for each pass with perfect body alignment. Feel your body in alignment as you make contact with the ball, and see the ball fly in the air and land exactly where you want it to land. What will you say to yourself before you set up for a pass that will help motivate you today/tonight? You want to think of something quick and easy to say, for instance; stay calm, I've got this, focus, smooth. Choose a phrase or word that works for you, and I want you to picture yourself setting up for a shot and saying this before each shot.

Now, take a moment to focus on form. Imagine yourself standing on the court. Your feet are planted on the gym floor, and your body is in alignment. You take your ready position, setting up to return a pass; feel yourself in perfect alignment and form. Watch as you perfectly execute a pass to your teammate. Then, watch as your teammate returns the pass perfectly, catching the opponent off guard. Your point!

Lastly, visualize a few key plays that you have discussed with your coach, and see yourself and your teammates acting out perfectly each play. Everyone is positioned correctly and working together, exactly how you planned. You execute each play with perfection and ease.

You are ready to play and ready to win. You are ready to show everyone what you are made of and how skilled your team is.

Remember to breathe. Stop and take five breaths if you need to at any point during the game.

Visualization Three

Breathing: Elephant Breath

Standing tall, take a big deep breath in as you raise your arms above you, and as you exhale, you let your arms swing between your legs like an elephant's trunk, letting the head and neck go. Roll up like a rag doll. Do this at least five times.

Visualize Your Game:

Imagine that your body is in tip-top condition today.

You feel great!

You are sending positive energy to all of your muscles and body parts.

Imagine and feel that everything is flowing, and you are ready physically for this game.

Imagine yourself entering the gym today and starting your warm-up.

Imagine your routine and what you will say to yourself to pump yourself up with positivity.

Imagine your warm-up going very well.

Now, imagine being on the court, and you are aware of the other people around you, and the people in the crowd. You can hear noises in the bleachers, but none of this matters to you because you are focusing your attention on hitting, serving, and playing.

295

Imagine all of your sets, bumps, and spikes being perfectly executed.

Imagine you serve with power, speed, and force.

Imagine your movement on the court to make each play is on point.

Feel your perfect form and flow while making successful passes.

You are in your zone, not letting distraction break your focus.

It feels natural and easy to make these plays.

Imagine setting up for your pass to a teammate with ease, focus, and determination.

You are now warmed up and ready to play at the top of your game!

You will let mistakes go easily and move on quickly.

You will let nothing stand in your way of playing great.

You will stay focused.

You will play the game you love to play!

When you are ready, you may open your eyes.

Visualization Four

Breathing Exercise:

Let's start out by bringing your attention to your breath. Let's see if you can focus on each inhale and each exhale. Can you notice where you are feeling your breath the most today? Do you feel the air moving in and out of your nostrils, or can you feel your chest rise and fall as you breathe, or maybe you notice your belly rising and falling as you breathe? Pick one of these three areas where you most naturally and easily feel your breath. Know that your breathing is always here for you as your anchor, grounding and stabilizing you when you need it.

Body Scan:

Next, allow your body to relax and soften. Starting at the top of your head, relax each body part as you work your way down your body. Allow the face to soften, the neck to relax, the shoulders to drop, the chest to release, and the arms and hands to relax. Move around to your back and allow this area to completely let go of tension; the hips begin to soften; the legs begin to release and elongate, and the feet and toes begin to let go. Your entire body should be completely relaxed and ready to focus on our visualization for today.

Set the Scene:

I want you to create a picture in your mind of the volleyball court you play on every day. Picture the details of this court, and imagine you are standing on the court admiring the scenery. Look around at the bleachers, the score board, and then the gym itself. This is the game that you love to play. You feel confident, important, and proud when you play this game. Take a moment to allow those great feelings, and the feelings of excitement to spread throughout your whole body.

Now, imagine you are getting ready to walk on the court with your teammates. You are pumped up, excited, eager, full of energy and positivity. You are ready to play this game and to play it well. Feel what it feels like, standing there with your team getting ready to walk out on that court. What do you notice? What can you hear? What can you see, people in the bleachers, coaches, players, friends? Soak it all in.

Now, you are ready to make your mark. You run onto the court and start your warm-up. Visualize your warm-up going smoothly and exactly the way you want it to. Take a moment to imagine feeling strong, fast, efficient, pumped up, and ready to play your best.

You know this game, your body knows this game, and your heart knows this game. You love to play, and you love to play well. Feel yourself getting into your zone where you are unstoppable, unbeatable, and unbreakable. Feel confident in your ability as a player, feel strong in your presence, feel grounded in your body and mind.

This is your moment to shine; this is your game to claim; this is your time to achieve success. Feel it, believe it, and allow it!

Bring your focus to your breathing. Notice the air coming into the nostrils and the air leaving the nostrils. Take one big deep breath in and release. When you are ready, you may open your eyes.

SOCCER VISUALIZATIONS

Visualization One

Breathing:

As we breathe today, I want you to say to yourself, "**I am confident**" each time you inhale and say to yourself, **"I am strong"** as you exhale. Continue to do this a few times, each time repeating I am confident on the inhale, and I am strong on the exhale. Allow yourself to settle in and get ready for this visualization.

Imagining A Positive Game:

Imagine walking onto the field, feeling confident, strong, and ready to perform well. See yourself walking with pep in your step, standing tall and proud, and feeling ready to take on this team.

Imagine yourself starting your warm-up.

What will you say to yourself when you are warming up? I am in control; I can do this; I will be a success; I am a great player?

Pick one of these affirmations, and repeat it to yourself right now three times silently.

See yourself warming-up and everything going the way you want it to. Feel the positive energy, the excitement, and the intense focus you have on getting and staying in your zone.

See yourself on the field, making smooth passes, handling the ball with grace and ease.

Feel your footwork and your quick, efficient moves as you dribble and pass the ball to your teammates. See the ball moving where you want it to move, feel the strength and quickness in your body, see yourself making shots on goal, and see the ball traveling through the air and hitting the net, making a goal.

Now, we will focus on what will happen during the game.

What will you say to yourself during the game to keep you motivated and focused?

Examples could be; stay focused, you got this, you know what you are doing, stay calm.

Pick one that works for you, and say this affirmation to yourself now, silently with conviction.

Take a moment to visualize what you want to happen today/tonight and how you want to play and perform. Imagine every play is executed with perfection. You are playing a flawless game, and your teammates are all on point. Everyone is in their zone and performing at their very best.

You are ready to play and ready to win. You are ready to show everyone what you are made of and how skilled your team is!

Bring your attention back to an inhalation and an exhalation.

When you are ready, you may open your eyes.

Visualization Two

Breathing: Heart and Belly Breathing

Place one hand on your heart and the other on your belly. Continue to breathe normally and naturally as you focus your attention on the pace of your breathing. You should notice that your breathing slows down when your hands are in this position. As you breathe, send kind wishes to yourself. You can say to yourself:

I am strong.
I am confident.
I am proud of who I am.
I am successful.
I am a winner!

After you repeat these affirmations to yourself, you may allow your hands to fall to your sides or rest in your lap.

We will begin the visualization now.

Recalling a Time:

I want you to remember when and why you wanted to play soccer. Can you remember this time? Can you picture the details? Where were you? Who were you with? What was going on around you? Let's take some time to recall this special time that you fell in love with this game and decided that you wanted to play soccer competitively. Soak in the memory and allow it to fill your mind's eye. Let the memory fill you up with joy, energy, positivity, and happiness.

Allow those positive feelings and feelings of determination, motivation, dedication, and drive to fill you up and spread to every part of your being. Soak up all of those wonderful feelings of the time when you first connected with the game. Now, try to take those wonderful feelings with you in today's game, and have fun playing this game.

Now, imagine being on the field right now. I want you to take three long, slow, deep breaths, in through the nose and out through the mouth. Stay in the moment with each breath you take.

You are ready to play today. You will use your breathing to help relax and calm yourself down if you feel you are getting too emotional or upset. You will turn your focus inward to get into your zone.

Now, take a moment to see yourself making shots on goal. Imagine making a few goals. Take a moment to visualize yourself dribbling the ball down the field, using your footwork to take on each defender, feel yourself in control of the ball, and then imagine taking your shot on goal and watching the ball successfully hit the net. Feel your body in alignment as you make each goal. Feel the ball make contact with your

303

foot, see the speed and line the ball is traveling as it enters the goal. What will you say to yourself before you try to score a goal or to defend a goal that will help motivate you today? You want to think of something quick and easy to say. For instance; I've got this, steady, stay in control, focus, smooth. Choose a phrase or word that works for you, and I want you to picture yourself setting up for a pass to a teammate, attempting a goal, or dribbling down the field and saying this before each play.

Now, take a moment to focus on dribbling. Imagine yourself on the field with the ball in your possession. See yourself dribbling the ball, looking for open teammates, and passing the ball efficiently, precisely and quickly. See the ball travel to your teammate with perfect speed and accuracy. Continue to imagine you and your teammates handling the ball with ease, making smooth, successful passes in order to score. Breathe and focus.

Next, visualize a few key plays that you have discussed with your coach, and see yourself and your teammates acting out perfectly each play. Everyone is positioned correctly and working together, exactly how you planned. You execute each play with perfection and ease.

You are ready to play and ready to win. You are ready to show everyone what you are made of and how skilled your team is!

Remember to breathe. Stop and take five breaths if you need to at any point during the game.

Visualization Three

Breathing: Elephant Breath

Standing tall, take a big deep breath in, as you raise your arms above you, and as you exhale, you let your arms swing between your legs like an elephant's trunk, letting the head and neck go. Roll up like a rag doll. Do this at least five times.

Visualize Your Game:

Imagine that your body is in tip-top condition today.

You feel great!

You are sending positive energy to all of your muscles and body parts.

Imagine and feel that everything is flowing, and you are ready physically for this game.

Imagine yourself entering the field today and starting your warm-up.

Imagine your routine and what you will say to yourself to pump yourself up with positivity.

Imagine your warm-up going very well.

Now, imagine being on the field, and you are aware of the other people around you, and the people in the crowd. You can hear noises on the field, but none of this matters to you because you are focusing your attention on passing, dribbling, and playing.

Imagine all of your passes being perfectly executed.

Imagine your movement on the field dribbling the ball is on point.

Feel your perfect form and flow while making successful passes and plays.

You are in your zone, not letting distractions break your focus.

It feels natural and easy to make these plays.

Imagine running on the field with ease, focus, and strength.

You are now warmed up and ready to play at the top of your game.

You will let mistakes go easily and move on quickly.

You will let nothing stand in your way of playing great.

You will stay focused.

You will play the game you love to play!

Bring your attention back to your breathing, focusing on an inhalation and an exhalation.

When you are ready, you may open your eyes.

Visualization Four

Breathing Exercise:

Let's start out by bringing your attention to your breath. Let's see if you can focus on each inhale and each exhale. Can you notice where you are feeling your breath the most today? Do you feel the air moving in and out of your nostrils, or can you feel your chest rise and fall as you breathe, or maybe you notice your belly rising and falling as you breathe? Pick one of these three areas where you most naturally and easily feel your breath. Know that your breathing is always here for you as your anchor, grounding and stabilizing you when you need it.

Body Scan:

Next, allow your body to relax and soften. Starting at the top of your head, relax each body part as you work your way down your body. Allow the face to soften, the neck to relax, the shoulders to drop, the chest to release, and the arms and hands to relax. Move around to your back and allow this area to completely let go of tension; the hips begin to soften; the legs begin to release and elongate, and the feet and toes begin to let go. Your entire body should be completely relaxed and ready to focus on our visualization for today.

Set the Scene:

I want you to create a picture in your mind of the soccer field you play on every day. Picture the details of this field, and imagine you are standing on the field admiring the scenery. Look around at the bleachers, the score board, and then the field itself. This is the game that you love to play. You feel confident, important, and proud when you play this game. Take a moment to allow those great feelings, and the feelings of excitement to spread throughout your whole body.

Now, imagine you are getting ready to enter the field with your teammates. You are pumped up, excited, eager, full of energy and positivity. You are ready to play this game and to play it well. Feel what it feels like, standing there with your team getting ready to enter the field. What do you notice? What can you hear? What can you see, people in the bleachers, coaches, players, friends? Soak it all in.

Now, you are ready to make your entrance. You run onto the field and start your warm-up. Visualize your warm-up going smoothly and exactly the way you want it to. Take a moment to imagine feeling strong, fast, efficient, pumped up, and ready to play your best.

You know this game, your body knows this game, and your heart knows this game. You love to play, and you love to play well. Feel yourself getting into your zone where you are unstoppable, unbeatable, and unbreakable. Feel confident in your ability as a player, feel strong in your presence, feel grounded in your body and mind.

This is your moment to shine; this is your game to claim; this is your time to achieve success. Feel it, believe it, and allow it!

Bring your focus to your breathing. Notice the air coming into the nostrils and the air leaving the nostrils. Take one big deep breath in and release. When you are ready, you may open your eyes.

FIELD HOCKEY
VISUALIZATIONS

Visualization One

Breathing:

As we breathe today, I want you to say to yourself, "**I am confident**" each time you inhale and say to yourself, **"I am strong"** as you exhale. Continue to do this a few times, each time repeating I am confident on the inhale, and I am strong on the exhale. Allow yourself to settle in and get ready for this visualization.

Imagining A Positive Game:

Imagine walking onto the field, feeling confident, strong, and ready to perform well. See yourself walking with pep in your step, standing tall and proud, and feeling ready to take on this team.

Imagine yourself starting your warm-up.

What will you say to yourself when you are warming up? I am in control; I can do this; I will be a success; I am a great player?

Pick one of these affirmations, and repeat it to yourself right now three times silently.

See yourself warming-up and everything going the way you want it to. Feel the positive energy, the excitement, and the intense focus you have on getting and staying in your zone.

See yourself on the field, making smooth passes, handling the ball and the stick with grace and ease. Feel your footwork and your quick, efficient moves as you jog down the field, driving and passing the ball to your teammates. See the ball moving where you want it to move, feel the strength and quickness in your body, see yourself making shots on goal, and see the ball hitting the net, making a goal.

Now, we will focus on what will happen during the game.

What will you say to yourself during the game to keep you motivated and focused?

Examples could be; stay focused, you got this, you know what you are doing, stay calm.

Pick one that works for you, and say this affirmation to yourself now, silently with conviction.

Take a moment to visualize what you want to happen today/tonight and how you want to play and perform. Imagine every play is executed with perfection. You are playing a flawless game, and your teammates are all on point. Everyone is in their zone and performing at their very best.

You are ready to play and ready to win. You are ready to show everyone what you are made of and how skilled your team is. Bring your attention back to an inhalation and an exhalation.

When you are ready, you may open your eyes.

Visualization Two

Breathing: Heart and Belly Breathing

Place one hand on your heart and the other on your belly. Continue to breathe normally and naturally as you focus your attention on the pace of your breathing. You should notice that your breathing slows down when your hands are in this position. As you breathe, send kind wishes to yourself. You can say to yourself:

I am strong.
I am confident.
I am proud of who I am.
I am successful.
I am a winner!

After you repeat these affirmations to yourself, you may allow your hands to fall to your sides or rest in your lap.

We will begin the visualization now.

Recalling a Time:

I want you to remember when and why you wanted to play field hockey. Can you remember this time? Can you picture the details? Where were you? Who were you with? What was going on around you? Take a moment to recall this special time that you fell in love with this game and decided that you wanted to play field hockey competitively. Soak in the memory and allow it to fill your mind's eye. Let the memory fill you up with joy, energy, positivity, and happiness.

Allow those positive feelings and feelings of determination, motivation, dedication, and drive to fill you up and spread to every part of your being. Soak up all of those wonderful feelings of the time when you first connected with the game. Now, try to take those wonderful feelings with you in today's game, and have fun playing this game.

Now, imagine being on the field right now. I want you to take three long, slow, deep breaths, in through the nose and out through the mouth. Stay in the moment with each breath you take.

You are ready to play today. You will use your breathing to help relax and calm yourself down if you feel you are getting too emotional or upset. You will turn your focus inward to get into your zone.

Now, take a moment to see yourself making shots on goal. Imagine making a few goals. Take a moment to visualize yourself working the ball down the field, using your footwork to take on each defender, feel yourself in control of the ball, and then imagine taking your shot on goal and watching the ball successfully hit the net. Feel your body in alignment as you make each goal. See your stick make perfect contact

313

with the ball, see the speed and line the ball is traveling as it enters the goal. What will you say to yourself before you try to score a goal or to defend a goal that will help motivate you today? You want to think of something quick and easy to say. For instance; I've got this, steady, stay in control, focus, smooth. Choose a phrase or word that works for you, and I want you to picture yourself setting up for a pass to a teammate, attempting a goal, or pushing the ball as you jog down the field and saying this before each play.

Now, take a moment to focus on ball control. Imagine yourself on the field with the ball in your possession. See yourself pushing and moving the ball down the field, looking for open teammates, and passing the ball efficiently, precisely and quickly. See the ball travel to your teammate with perfect speed and accuracy. Continue to imagine you and your teammates handling the ball with ease, making smooth, successful passes in order to score. Breathe and focus.

Next, visualize a few key plays that you have discussed with your coach, and see yourself and your teammates acting out perfectly each play. Everyone is positioned correctly and working together, exactly how you planned. You execute each play with perfection and ease.

You are ready to play and ready to win. You are ready to show everyone what you are made of and how skilled your team is!

Remember to breathe. Stop and take five breaths if you need to at any point during the game

Visualization Three

Breathing: Elephant Breath

Standing tall, take a big deep breath in, as you raise your arms above you, and as you exhale, you let your arms swing between your legs like an elephant's trunk, letting the head and neck go. Roll up like a rag doll. Do this at least five times.

Visualize Your Game:

Imagine that your body is in tip-top condition today.

You feel great!

You are sending positive energy to all of your muscles and body parts.

Imagine and feel that everything is flowing, and you are ready physically for this game.

Imagine yourself entering the field today and starting your warm-up.

Imagine your routine and what you will say to yourself to pump yourself up with positivity.

Imagine your warm-up going very well.

Now, imagine being on the field, and you are aware of the other people around you, and the people in the crowd. You can hear noises on the field, but none of this matters to you because you are focusing your attention on passing, pushing, and driving the ball down the field, and playing.

Imagine all of your passes being perfectly executed.

Imagine your movement on the field handling the ball is on point.

Feel your perfect form and flow while making successful passes and plays.

You are in your zone, not letting distractions break your focus.

It feels natural and easy to make these plays.

Imagine running on the field with ease, focus, and strength.

You are now warmed up and ready to play at the top of your game.

You will let mistakes go easily and move on quickly.

You will let nothing stand in your way of playing great.

You will stay focused.

You will play the game you love to play!

Bring your attention back to your breathing, focusing on an inhalation and an exhalation.

When you are ready, you may open your eyes.

Visualization Four

Breathing Exercise:

Let's start out by bringing your attention to your breath. Let's see if you can focus on each inhale and each exhale. Can you notice where you are feeling your breath the most today? Do you feel the air moving in and out of your nostrils, or can you feel your chest rise and fall as you breathe, or maybe you notice your belly rising and falling as you breathe? Pick one of these three areas where you most naturally and easily feel your breath. Know that your breathing is always here for you as your anchor, grounding and stabilizing you when you need it.

Body Scan:

Next, allow your body to relax and soften. Starting at the top of your head, relax each body part as you work your way down your body. Allow the face to soften, the neck to relax, the shoulders to drop, the chest to release, and the arms and hands to relax. Move around to your back and allow this area to completely let go of tension; the hips begin to soften; the legs begin to release and elongate, and the feet and toes begin to let go. Your entire body should be completely relaxed and ready to focus on our visualization for today.

Set the Scene:

I want you to create a picture in your mind of the field hockey field you play on every day. Picture the details of this field, and imagine you are standing on the field admiring the scenery. Look around at the bleachers, the score board, and then the field itself. This is the game that you love to play. You feel confident, important, and proud when you play this game. Take a moment to allow those great feelings, and the feelings of excitement to spread throughout your whole body.

Now, imagine you are getting ready to enter the field with your teammates. You are pumped up, excited, eager, full of energy and positivity. You are ready to play this game and to play it well. Feel what it feels like, standing there with your team getting ready to enter the field. What do you notice? What can you hear? What can you see, people in the bleachers, coaches, players, friends? Soak it all in.

Now, you are ready to make your entrance. You run onto the field and start your warm-up. Visualize your warm-up going smoothly and exactly the way you want it to. Take a moment to imagine feeling strong, fast, efficient, pumped up, and ready to play your best.

You know this game, your body knows this game, and your heart knows this game. You love to play, and you love to play well. Feel yourself getting into your zone where you are unstoppable, unbeatable, and unbreakable. Feel confident in your ability as a player, feel strong in your presence, feel grounded in your body and mind.

This is your moment to shine; this is your game to claim; this is your time to achieve success. Feel it, believe it, and allow it!

Bring your focus to your breathing. Notice the air coming into the nostrils and the air leaving the nostrils. Take one big deep breath in and release. When you are ready, you may open your eyes.

CROSS-COUNTRY/ TRACK VISUALIZATIONS

Visualization One

Breathing:

As we breathe today, I want you to say to yourself, "**I am confident**" each time you inhale and say to yourself, "**I am strong**" as you exhale. Continue to do this a few times, each time repeating I am confident on the inhale, and I am strong on the exhale. Allow yourself to settle in and get ready for this visualization.

Imagining A Positive Meet:

Imagine walking onto the track, feeling confident, strong, and ready to perform well. See yourself walking with pep in your step, standing tall and proud, and feeling ready to run your best run, perform your best event, and take on this team.

Imagine yourself starting your warm-up.

What will you say to yourself when you are warming up? I am fast and efficient; I can do this; I will be a success; I am great at what I do?

Pick one of these affirmations, and repeat it to yourself right now three times silently.

See yourself warming-up and everything going the way you want it to. Feel the positive energy, the excitement, and the intense focus you have on getting and staying in your zone.

See yourself on the track, stretching, and warming your body up for your race or event. Feel your quickness, speed, accuracy as you jog on the track, and focus on your perfect form. Feel your rhythm; your arms are swinging and pumping quickly, your body is in an upright position, your legs moving quickly, and your leg stride is driving you forward around the track. You are focused and feeling strong.

Now, we will focus on what will happen during your race or event.

What will you say to yourself during your race to keep you motivated and focused?

Examples could be; stay focused, you got this, you know what you are doing, fast and efficient strides, stay calm.

Pick one that works for you, and say this affirmation to yourself now, silently with conviction.

Take a moment to visualize what you want to happen today and how you want to perform. Imagine every move you make is executed with perfection. You are running a flawless race. Everyone on your team is in their zone and performing at their very best.

You are ready to perform and ready to win. You are ready to show everyone what you are made of and how skilled your team is!

Bring your attention back to an inhalation and an exhalation.

When you are ready, you may open your eyes.

Visualization Two

Breathing: Heart and Belly Breathing

Place one hand on your heart and the other on your belly. Continue to breathe normally and naturally as you focus your attention on the pace of your breathing. You should notice that your breathing slows down when your hands are in this position. As you breathe, send kind wishes to yourself. You can say to yourself:

I am strong.
I am confident.
I am proud of who I am.
I am successful.
I am a winner!

After you repeat these affirmations to yourself, you may allow your hands to fall to your sides or rest in your lap.

We will begin the visualization now.

Recalling a Time:

I want you to remember when and why you wanted to join track. Can you remember this time? Can you picture the details? Where were you? Who were you with? What was going on around you? Take a moment to recall this special time that you fell in love with this sport and decided that you wanted to race competitively. Soak in the memory and allow it to fill your mind's eye. Let the memory fill you up with joy, energy, positivity, and happiness.

Allow those positive feelings and feelings of determination, motivation, dedication, and drive to fill you up and spread to every part of your being. Soak up all of those wonderful feelings of the time when you first connected with this sport. Now, try to take those wonderful feelings with you in today's competition, and have fun participating in this sport.

Now, imagine being on the track right now. I want you to take three long, slow, deep breaths, in through the nose and out through the mouth. Stay in the moment with each breath you take.

You are ready to perform today. You will use your breathing to help relax and calm yourself down if you feel you are getting nervous. You will turn your focus inward to get into your zone.

Now, take a moment to see yourself running the perfect race, or executing your event with precision. Imagine taking over the competition. Visualize yourself running with perfect form and flow, leading the pack, feeling calm and confident in your ability to win this race. What will you say to yourself before you begin your race/event that will help motivate you today? You want to think of something quick and easy to say, for instance; I've got this, I am fast and strong, stay calm and cool, focus, smooth. Choose a phrase or word that works for you, and I want you to picture yourself in your ready position before your race or event, and saying this before the gun goes off.

Now, visualize a few key strategies you have discussed with your coach, and see yourself using these tips during your performance. You execute each move with perfection and ease.

You are ready to perform and ready to win. You are ready to show everyone what you are made of and how skilled your team is!

Remember to breathe. Stop and take five breaths if you need to at any point during the meet.

Visualization Three

Breathing: Elephant Breath

Standing tall, take a big deep breath in, as you raise your arms above you, and as you exhale, you let your arms swing between your legs like an elephant's trunk, letting the head and neck go. Roll up like a rag doll. Do this at least five times.

Visualize Your Meet:

Imagine that your body is in tip-top condition today.

You feel great!

You are sending positive energy to all of your muscles and body parts.

Imagine and feel that everything is flowing, and you are ready physically for this competition.

Imagine yourself entering on the track today and starting your warm-up.

Imagine your routine and what you will say to yourself to pump yourself up with positivity.

Imagine your warm-up going very well.

Now imagine being on the track, and you are aware of the other people around you, and the people in the crowd. You can hear noises on the field, but none of this matters to you because you are focusing your attention on running, stretching, and warming up.

Imagine your movements are on point.
Feel your perfect form and flow while warming up.
You are in your zone, not letting distractions break your focus.
It feels natural and easy for you to perform.
Imagine running on the track with ease, focus, and strength.
You are now warmed up and ready to perform at the top of your game.
You will let mistakes go easily and move on quickly.
You will let nothing stand in your way of performing well.
You will stay focused.
You will succeed in the sport you love!
Bring your attention back to your breathing, focusing on an inhalation and an exhalation.
When you are ready, you may open your eyes.

Visualization Four

Breathing Exercise:

Let's start out by bringing your attention to your breath. Let's see if you can focus on each inhale and each exhale. Can you notice where you are feeling your breath the most today? Do you feel the air moving in and out of your nostrils, or can you feel your chest rise and fall as you breathe, or maybe you notice your belly rising and falling as you breathe? Pick one of these three areas where you most naturally and easily feel your breath. Know that your breathing is always here for you as your anchor, grounding and stabilizing you when you need it.

Body Scan:

Next, allow your body to relax and soften. Starting at the top of your head, relax each body part as you work your way down your body. Allow the face to soften, the neck to relax, the shoulders to drop, the chest to release, and the arms and hands to relax. Move around to your back and allow this area to completely let go of tension; the hips begin to soften; the legs begin to release and elongate, and the feet and toes begin to let go. Your entire body should be completely relaxed and ready to focus on our visualization for today.

Set the Scene:

I want you to create a picture in your mind of the track you practice on every day. Picture the details of this track, and imagine you are standing on the track admiring the scenery. Look around at the bleachers, the score board, the field, and the track itself. This is the sport that you love to be a part of. You feel confident, important, and proud when you compete. Take a moment to allow those great feelings, and the feelings of excitement to spread throughout your whole body.

Now, imagine you are getting ready to enter the track with your teammates. You are pumped up, excited, eager, full of energy and positivity. You are ready to compete and perform well. Feel what it feels like, standing there with your team getting ready to enter the track. What do you notice? What can you hear? What can you see, people in the bleachers, coaches, teammates, friends? Soak it all in.

Now, you are ready to make your entrance. You run onto the track and start your warm-up. Visualize your warm-up going smoothly and exactly the way you want it to. Take a moment to imagine feeling strong, fast, efficient, pumped up, and ready to perform at your best.

You know this sport, your body knows this sport, and your heart knows this sport. You love to perform, and you love to perform well. Feel yourself getting into your zone where you are unstoppable, unbeatable, and unbreakable. Feel confident in your ability as an athlete, feel strong in your presence, feel grounded in your body and mind.

This is your moment to shine; this is your event to claim; this is your time to achieve success. Feel it, believe it, and allow it!

Bring your focus to your breathing. Notice the air coming into the nostrils and the air leaving the nostrils. Take one big deep breath in and release. When you are ready, you may open your eyes.

WRESTLING VISUALIZATIONS

Visualization One

Breathing:

As we breathe today, I want you to say to yourself, "**I am confident**" each time you inhale and say to yourself, **"I am strong"** as you exhale. Continue to do this a few times, each time repeating I am confident on the inhale, and I am strong on the exhale. Allow yourself to settle in and get ready for this visualization.

Imagining A Positive Match:

Imagine walking into the gym, feeling confident, strong, and ready to perform well. See yourself walking with pep in your step, standing tall and proud, and feeling ready to have your best match, perform at your best, and take on this team.

Imagine yourself starting your warm-up on the mats.

What will you say to yourself when you are warming up? I am confident; I can do this; I am a success; I am great at what I do?

Pick one of these affirmations and repeat it to yourself right now three times silently.

See yourself warming-up and everything going the way you want it to. Feel the positive energy, the excitement, and the intense focus you have on getting and staying in your zone.

See yourself on the mats, practicing your moves, holds, and body positions, warming your body up for your match. Feel your smoothness, accuracy, and perfect form as you practice trying to pin, and take-down your teammate. Feel your rhythm; your feet never stop moving; you are focused on your breathing to give you energy; you are getting ready to pin your opponent; and you are always ready for your escape move. You are focused and feeling strong.

Now, we will focus on what will happen during your match.

What will you say to yourself during your match to keep you motivated and focused?

Examples could be; stay focused, you got this, you are strong, stay calm and breathe.

Pick one that works for you, and say this affirmation to yourself now, silently with conviction.

Take a moment to visualize what you want to happen today and how you want to perform. Imagine every takedown is executed with perfection. You are wrestling a flawless match. Every stance you take, every position you are in, and every move you make goes exactly the way you want it to. Your attack shots are on point. Visualize a single-leg takedown, and a double-leg takedown being perfectly executed.

You are ready to perform and ready to win. You are ready to show everyone what you are made of and how skilled your team is!

Bring your attention back to an inhalation and an exhalation.

When you are ready, you may open your eyes.

Visualization Two

Breathing: Heart and Belly Breathing

Place one hand on your heart and the other on your belly. Continue to breathe normally and naturally as you focus your attention on the pace of your breathing. You should notice that your breathing slows down when your hands are in this position. As you breathe, send kind wishes to yourself. You can say to yourself:

I am strong.
I am confident.
I am proud of who I am.
I am successful.
I am a winner!

After you repeat these affirmations to yourself, you may allow your hands to fall to your sides or rest in your lap.

We will begin the visualization now.

Recalling a Time:

I want you to remember when and why you wanted to wrestle. Can you remember this time? Can you picture the details? Where were you? Who were you with? What was going on around you? Take a moment to recall this special time that you fell in love with wrestling and decided that you wanted to wrestle competitively. Soak in the memory and allow it to fill your mind's eye. Let the memory fill you up with joy, energy, positivity, and happiness.

Allow those positive feelings and feelings of determination, motivation, dedication, and drive to fill you up and spread to every part of your being. Soak up all of those wonderful feelings of the time when you first connected with this sport. Now, try to take those wonderful feelings with you in today's match, and have fun participating in this sport.

Now, imagine being on the mat right now. I want you to take three long, slow, deep breaths, in through the nose and out through the mouth. Stay in the moment with each breath you take.

You are ready to wrestle today. You will use your breathing to help relax and calm yourself down if you feel you are getting nervous. You will turn your focus inward to get into your zone.

Now, take a moment to see yourself wrestling a perfect match. Imagine being on top the entire match. Visualize yourself attacking your opponent with precision and accuracy. Your defense and escape techniques are easy for you to maneuver. Imagine lifting and pinning your opponent with ease. What will you say to yourself before you begin your match that will help motivate you today? You want to think of something quick and easy to say, for instance; I've got this, I know this sport well, stay calm and cool, focus, stay strong. Choose a phrase or word that works for you, and I want you to picture yourself on the mat before your match and saying this to yourself before your match begins.

You are ready to perform and ready to win. You are ready to show everyone what you are made of and how skilled your team is!

Remember to breathe. Stop and take five breaths if you need to at any point during the match.

Visualization Three

Breathing: Elephant Breath

Standing tall, take a big deep breath in, as you raise your arms above you, and as you exhale, you let your arms swing between your legs like an elephant's trunk, letting the head and neck go. Roll up like a rag doll. Do this at least five times.

Visualize Your Match:

Imagine that your body is in tip-top condition today.

You feel great!

You are sending positive energy to all of your muscles and body parts.

Imagine and feel that everything is flowing, and you are ready physically for this match.

Imagine yourself on the mat today and starting your warm-up.

Imagine your routine and what you will say to yourself to pump yourself up with positivity.

Imagine your warm-up going very well.

Now, imagine being on the mat, and you are aware of the other people around you, and the people in the crowd. You can hear noises coming from spectators, but none of this matters to you, because you are focusing your attention on defending, attacking, and warming up.

Imagine your moves feel smooth and strong.
Feel your perfect form and flow while warming up.
Your footwork and agility are on point and accurate. Your movement on the mat is quick.
You are in your zone, not letting distractions break your focus.
It feels natural and easy for you to perform.
Imagine wrestling with ease, focus, and strength.
You are now warmed up and ready to perform at the top of your game.
You will let mistakes go easily and move on quickly.
You will let nothing stand in your way of performing well.
You will stay focused.
You will succeed in the sport you love!
Bring your attention back to your breathing, focusing on an inhalation and an exhalation.
When you are ready, you may open your eyes.

Visualization Four

Breathing Exercise:

Let's start out by bringing your attention to your breath. Let's see if you can focus on each inhale and each exhale. Can you notice where you are feeling your breath the most today? Do you feel the air moving in and out of your nostrils, or can you feel your chest rise and fall as you breathe, or maybe you notice your belly rising and falling as you breathe? Pick one of these three areas where you most naturally and easily feel your breath. Know that your breathing is always here for you as your anchor, grounding and stabilizing you when you need it.

Body Scan:

Next, allow your body to relax and soften. Starting at the top of your head, relax each body part as you work your way down your body. Allow the face to soften, the neck to relax, the shoulders to drop, the chest to release, and the arms and hands to relax. Move around to your back and allow this area to completely let go of tension; the hips begin to soften; the legs begin to release and elongate, and the feet and toes begin to let go. Your entire body should be completely relaxed and ready to focus on our visualization for today.

Set the Scene:

I want you to create a picture in your mind of the gym you practice in every day. Picture the details of this gym, and imagine you are standing on the mats admiring the scenery. You notice the bleachers, the score board, the clock, and the entire gym itself. You feel confident, important, and proud when you compete. Take a moment to allow those great feelings, and the feelings of excitement to spread throughout your whole body.

Now, imagine you are getting ready to enter the gym with your teammates. You are pumped up, excited, eager, full of energy, and positivity. You are ready to compete and perform well.

Now, you are ready to make your entrance. You walk in the gym with your teammates, and you are ready to start your warm-up. Visualize your warm-up going smoothly and exactly the way you want it to. Your body feels loose, relaxed, and ready to wrestle. Take a moment to imagine feeling strong, efficient, precise, and ready to perform at your best.

You know this sport, your body knows this sport, and your heart knows this sport. You love to wrestle, and you love to wrestle well. Feel yourself getting into your zone where you are unstoppable, unbeatable, and unbreakable. Feel confident in your ability as an athlete, feel strong in your presence, feel grounded in your body and mind.

This is your moment to shine; this is your match to claim; this is your time to achieve success. Feel it, believe it, and allow it!

Bring your focus to your breathing. Notice the air coming into the nostrils and the air leaving the nostrils. Take one big deep breath in and release. When you are ready, you may open your eyes.

SWIMMING VISUALIZATIONS

Visualization One

Breathing:

As we breathe today, I want you to say to yourself, **"I am confident"** each time you inhale and say to yourself, **"I am strong"** as you exhale. Continue to do this a few times, each time repeating I am confident on the inhale, and I am strong on the exhale. Allow yourself to settle in and get ready for this visualization.

Imagining A Positive Race:

Imagine walking onto the pool deck, feeling confident, strong, and ready to perform well. See yourself walking with pep in your step, standing tall and proud, and feeling ready to swim your best race, perform your best event, and take on this team.

Imagine yourself starting your warm-up.

What will you say to yourself when you are warming up? I am fast and efficient; I can do this; I am a success; I am great at what I do?

Pick one of these affirmations, and repeat it to yourself right now three times silently.

See yourself warming-up and everything going the way you want it to. Feel the positive energy, the excitement, and the intense focus you have on getting and staying in your zone.

See yourself in the pool, gliding through the water, warming your body up for your race. Feel your quickness, speed, accuracy, and perfect form as you swim your stroke, and perform your flip turns. Feel your rhythm; your arms gliding through the water, your legs kicking with strength and power; and your breathing is effortless. You are focused and feeling strong.

Now, we will focus on what will happen during your race.

What will you say to yourself during your race to keep you motivated and focused?

Examples could be; stay focused, you got this, glide, you are strong, stay calm.

Pick one that works for you, and say this affirmation to yourself now, silently with conviction.

Take a moment to visualize what you want to happen today and how you want to perform. Imagine every stroke you take is executed with perfection. You are swimming a flawless race. Everyone on your team is in their zone and performing at their very best as well.

You are ready to perform and ready to win. You are ready to show everyone what you are made of and how skilled your team is!

Bring your attention back to an inhalation and an exhalation.

When you are ready, you may open your eyes.

Visualization Two

Breathing: Heart and Belly Breathing

Place one hand on your heart and the other on your belly. Continue to breathe normally and naturally as you focus your attention on the pace of your breathing. You should notice that your breathing slows down when your hands are in this position. As you breathe, send kind wishes to yourself. You can say to yourself:

I am strong.
I am confident.
I am proud of who I am.
I am successful.
I am a winner!

After you repeat these affirmations to yourself, you may allow your hands to fall to your sides or rest in your lap.

We will begin the visualization now.

Recalling a Time:

I want you to remember when and why you wanted to swim. Can you remember this time? Can you picture the details? Where were you? Who were you with? What was going on around you? Take a moment to recall this special time that you fell in love with swimming and decided that you wanted to swim competitively. Soak in the memory and allow it to fill your mind's eye. Let the memory fill you up with joy, energy, positivity, and happiness.

Allow those positive feelings and feelings of determination, motivation, dedication, and drive to fill you up and spread to every part of your being. Soak up all of those wonderful feelings of the time when you first connected with this sport. Now, try to take those wonderful feelings with you in today's competition, and have fun participating in this sport.

Now, imagine being in the pool right now. I want you to take three long, slow, deep breaths, in through the nose and out through the mouth. Stay in the moment with each breath you take.

You are ready to perform today. You will use your breathing to help relax and calm yourself down if you feel you are getting nervous. You will turn your focus inward to get into your zone.

Now, take a moment to see yourself swimming the perfect race. Visualize yourself diving off the block before anyone else, entering into the water, feeling the coolness of the water, and taking your first stroke ahead of the competition. Imagine taking the lead instantly and feeling strong. Visualize yourself swimming with perfect form and flow, leading the pack, feeling calm and confident in your ability to win this race. What will you say to yourself before you begin your race that will help motivate you today? You want to think of something quick and easy to say, for instance; I've got this, I am fast and strong, stay calm and cool, focus, smooth. Choose a phrase or word that works for you, and I want you to picture yourself on the starting block before your race and saying this before the gun goes off.

You are ready to perform and ready to win. You are ready to show everyone what you are made of and how skilled your team is!

Remember to breathe. Stop and take five breaths if you need to at any point during the meet.

Visualization Three

Breathing: Elephant Breath

Standing tall, take a big deep breath in, as you raise your arms above you, and as you exhale, you let your arms swing between your legs like an elephant's trunk, letting the head and neck go. Roll up like a rag doll. Do this at least five times.

Visualize Your Meet:

Imagine that your body is in tip-top condition today.

You feel great!

You are sending positive energy to all of your muscles and body parts.

Imagine and feel that everything is flowing, and you are ready physically for this competition.

Imagine yourself entering the pool today and starting your warm-up.

Imagine your routine and what you will say to yourself to pump yourself up with positivity.

Imagine your warm-up going very well.

Now, imagine being on the pool deck, and you are aware of the other people around you, and the people in the crowd. You can hear noises coming from the stands, but none of this matters to you, because you are focusing your attention on swimming, stretching, and warming up.

Imagine your movements are on point.
Feel your perfect form and flow while warming up.
You are in your zone, not letting distractions break your focus.
It feels natural and easy for you to perform.
Imagine swimming with ease, focus, and strength.
You are now warmed up and ready to perform at the top of your game.
You will let mistakes go easily and move on quickly.
You will let nothing stand in your way of performing well.
You will stay focused.
You will succeed in the sport you love!
Bring your attention back to your breathing, focusing on an inhalation and an exhalation.
When you are ready, you may open your eyes.

Visualization Four

Breathing Exercise:

Let's start out by bringing your attention to your breath. Let's see if you can focus on each inhale and each exhale. Can you notice where you are feeling your breath the most today? Do you feel the air moving in and out of your nostrils, or can you feel your chest rise and fall as you breathe, or maybe you notice your belly rising and falling as you breathe? Pick one of these three areas where you most naturally and easily feel your breath. Know that your breathing is always here for you as your anchor, grounding and stabilizing you when you need it.

Body Scan:

Next, allow your body to relax and soften. Starting at the top of your head, relax each body part as you work your way down your body. Allow the face to soften, the neck to relax, the shoulders to drop, the chest to release, and the arms and hands to relax. Move around to your back and allow this area to completely let go of tension; the hips begin to soften; the legs begin to release and elongate, and the feet and toes begin to let go. Your entire body should be completely relaxed and ready to focus on our visualization for today.

Set the Scene:

I want you to create a picture in your mind of the pool you practice in every day. Picture the details of this pool, and imagine you are standing on the pool deck admiring the scenery. Look around at the stands, the clock, the pool deck, and the pool itself. This is the sport that you love to be a part of. You feel confident, important, and proud when you compete. Take a moment to allow those great feelings, and the feelings of excitement to spread throughout your whole body.

Now, imagine you are getting ready to enter the pool with your teammates. You are pumped up, excited, eager, full of energy and positivity. You are ready to compete and perform well. Feel what it feels like, standing there with your team getting ready to enter the pool. What do you notice? What can you hear? What can you see, people in the stands, coaches, teammates, friends? Soak it all in.

Now, you are ready to make your entrance. You walk onto the pool deck, get changed, and you are ready to start your warm-up. Visualize your warm-up going smoothly and exactly the way you want it to. Take a moment to imagine feeling strong, fast, efficient, pumped up, and ready to perform at your best. The water is the perfect temperature and you can't wait to swim!

You know this sport, your body knows this sport, and your heart knows this sport. You love to swim, and you love to swim well. Feel yourself getting into your zone where you are unstoppable, unbeatable, and unbreakable. Feel confident in your ability as an athlete, feel strong in your presence, feel grounded in your body and mind.

This is your moment to shine; this is your event to claim; this is your time to achieve success. Feel it, believe it, and allow it!

Bring your focus to your breathing. Notice the air coming into the nostrils and the air leaving the nostrils. Take one big deep breath in and release. When you are ready, you may open your eyes.

GOLF VISUALIZATIONS

Visualization One

Breathing:

As we breathe today, I want you to say to yourself, "**I am confident**" each time you inhale and say to yourself, **"I am strong"** as you exhale. Continue to do this a few times, each time repeating I am confident on the inhale, and I am strong on the exhale. Allow yourself to settle in and get ready for this visualization.

Imagining A Positive Match:

Imagine walking onto the golf course, feeling confident, strong, and ready to perform well. See yourself walking with pep in your step, standing tall and proud, and feeling ready to golf your best game, perform at your best, and take on this team.

Imagine yourself starting your warm-up on the range.

What will you say to yourself when you are warming up? I am confident; I can do this; I am a success; I am great at what I do?

Pick one of these affirmations, and repeat it to yourself right now three times silently.

See yourself warming-up and everything going the way you want it to. Feel the positive energy, the excitement, and the intense focus you have on getting and staying in your zone.

See yourself on the range, taking practice shot after practice shot, warming your body up for your match. Feel your smoothness, accuracy, and perfect form as you swing the club each time. Feel your rhythm; your arms are loose and relaxed; your grip is firm; your stance is strong and solid; and your swing is effortless and precise. You hit your drives smooth, long, and straight. Your iron shots are precise and accurate. You are focused and feeling strong.

Now, we will focus on what will happen during your game.

What will you say to yourself during your round to keep you motivated and focused?

Examples could be; stay focused, you got this, you are strong, stay calm.

Pick one that works for you, and say this affirmation to yourself now, silently with conviction.

Take a moment to visualize what you want to happen today and how you want to perform. Imagine every stroke you take is executed with perfection. You are golfing a flawless round. Every shot you take goes exactly where you want it to. Everyone on your team is in their zone and performing at their very best as well.

You are ready to perform and ready to win. You are ready to show everyone what you are made of and how skilled your team is!

Bring your attention back to an inhalation and an exhalation.

When you are ready, you may open your eyes.

Visualization Two

Breathing: Heart and Belly Breathing

Place one hand on your heart and the other on your belly. Continue to breathe normally and naturally as you focus your attention on the pace of your breathing. You should notice that your breathing slows down when your hands are in this position. As you breathe, send kind wishes to yourself. You can say to yourself:

I am strong.
I am confident.
I am proud of who I am.
I am successful.
I am a winner!

After you repeat these affirmations to yourself, you may allow your hands to fall to your sides or rest in your lap.

We will begin the visualization now.

Recalling a Time:

I want you to remember when and why you wanted to play golf. Can you remember this time? Can you picture the details? Where were you? Who were you with? What was going on around you? Take a moment to recall this special time that you fell in love with golf and decided that you wanted to golf competitively. Soak in the memory and allow it to fill your mind's eye. Let the memory fill you up with joy, energy, positivity, and happiness.

Allow those positive feelings and feelings of determination, motivation, dedication, and drive to fill you up and spread to every part of your being. Soak up all of those wonderful feelings of the time when you first connected with this sport. Now, try to take those wonderful feelings with you in today's competition, and have fun participating in this sport.

Now, imagine being on the course right now. I want you to take three long, slow, deep breaths, in through the nose and out through the mouth. Stay in the moment with each breath you take.

You are ready to play today. You will use your breathing to help relax and calm yourself down if you feel you are getting nervous. You will turn your focus inward to get into your zone.

Now, take a moment to see yourself golfing a perfect, bogie free round. Imagine being in the lead the entire round. Visualize yourself swinging the club with perfect form and flow, feeling calm and confident in your ability to win this match. What will you say to yourself before you begin your match that will help motivate you today? You want to think of something quick and easy to say, for instance; I've got this, I know this game well, stay calm and cool, focus, smooth swing. Choose a phrase or word that works for you, and I want you to picture yourself on the first tee before your match, and saying this to yourself before you tee off.

You are ready to perform and ready to win. You are ready to show everyone what you are made of and how skilled your team is!

Remember to breathe. Stop and take five breaths if you need to at any point during the round.

Visualization Three

Breathing: Elephant Breath

Standing tall, take a big deep breath in, as you raise your arms above you, and as you exhale, you let your arms swing between your legs like an elephant's trunk, letting the head and neck go. Roll up like a rag doll. Do this at least five times.

Visualize Your Game:

Imagine that your body is in tip-top condition today.

You feel great!

You are sending positive energy to all of your muscles and body parts.

Imagine and feel that everything is flowing, and you are ready physically for this match.

Imagine yourself on the range today and starting your warm-up.

Imagine your routine and what you will say to yourself to pump yourself up with positivity.

Imagine your warm-up going very well.

Now, imagine being on the practice putting green, and you are aware of the other people around you, and the people in the crowd. You can hear soft voices coming from spectators, but none of this matters to you, because you are focusing your attention on putting, chipping, and warming up.

Imagine your swing feels smooth and strong. Every putt is dropping, one after the other. Your ability to read the green is on point, and your stroke is even and steady.

Feel your perfect form and flow while warming up.
You are in your zone, not letting distractions break your focus.
It feels natural and easy for you to perform.
Imagine swinging with ease, focus, and strength.
You are now warmed up and ready to perform at the top of your game.
You will let mistakes go easily and move on quickly.
You will let nothing stand in your way of performing well.
You will stay focused.
You will succeed in the sport you love!
Bring your attention back to your breathing, focusing on an inhalation and an exhalation.
When you are ready, you may open your eyes.

Visualization Four

Breathing Exercise:

Let's start out by bringing your attention to your breath. Let's see if you can focus on each inhale and each exhale. Can you notice where you are feeling your breath the most today? Do you feel the air moving in and out of your nostrils, or can you feel your chest rise and fall as you breathe, or maybe you notice your belly rising and falling as you breathe? Pick one of these three areas where you most naturally and easily feel your breath. Know that your breathing is always here for you as your anchor, grounding and stabilizing you when you need it.

Body Scan:

Next, allow your body to relax and soften. Starting at the top of your head, relax each body part as you work your way down your body. Allow the face to soften, the neck to relax, the shoulders to drop, the chest to release, and the arms and hands to relax. Move around to your back and allow this area to completely let go of tension; the hips begin to soften; the legs begin to release and elongate, and the feet and toes begin to let go. Your entire body should be completely relaxed and ready to focus on our visualization for today.

Set the Scene:

I want you to create a picture in your mind of the golf course you practice on every day. Picture the details of this course, and imagine you are standing on the first tee admiring the scenery. Look around at the beautifully manicured fairways, the lush greens, the trees that line the fairways, the flag stick on the first green, and the clubhouse. You love to be able to play this sport outdoors, with such beautiful surroundings. How lucky are you? You feel confident, important, and proud when you compete. Take a moment to allow those great feelings, and the feelings of excitement to spread throughout your whole body.

Now, imagine you are getting ready to enter the golf course with your teammates. You are pumped up, excited, eager, full of energy, and positivity. You are ready to compete and perform well.

Now, you are ready to make your entrance. You walk over to the driving range, and you are ready to start your warm-up. Visualize your warm-up going smoothly and exactly the way you want it to. Your body feels loose, relaxed, and ready to play a great round of golf. Take a moment to imagine feeling strong, efficient, precise, and ready to perform at your best.

You know this sport, your body knows this sport, and your heart knows this sport. You love to golf, and you love to golf well. Feel yourself getting into your zone where you are unstoppable, unbeatable, and unbreakable. Feel confident in your ability as an athlete, feel strong in your presence, feel grounded in your body and mind.

This is your moment to shine; this is your round to claim; this is your time to achieve success. Feel it, believe it, and allow it!

Bring your focus to your breathing. Notice the air coming into the nostrils and the air leaving the nostrils. Take one big deep breath in and release. When you are ready, you may open your eyes.

TENNIS VISUALIZATIONS

Visualization One

Breathing:

As we breathe today, I want you to say to yourself, **"I am confident"** each time you inhale and say to yourself, **"I am strong"** as you exhale. Continue to do this a few times, each time repeating I am confident on the inhale, and I am strong on the exhale. Allow yourself to settle in and get ready for this visualization.

Imagining A Positive Match:

Imagine walking onto the tennis courts, feeling confident, strong, and ready to perform well. See yourself walking with pep in your step, standing tall and proud, and feeling ready to play your best game, perform at your best, and take on this team.

Imagine yourself starting your warm-up on the court.

What will you say to yourself when you are warming up? I am confident; I can do this; I am a success; I am great at what I do?

Pick one of these affirmations and repeat it to yourself right now three times silently.

See yourself warming-up and everything going the way you want it to. Feel the positive energy, the excitement, and the intense focus you have on getting and staying in your zone.

See yourself on the court, practicing your forehand and backhand shots, warming your body up for your match. Feel your smoothness, accuracy, and perfect form as you swing your racket each time. Feel your rhythm; your arms are loose and relaxed; your grip is firm; your stance is strong and solid; and your swing is effortless and precise. Now, imagine getting ready to serve. As you throw the ball in the air, your eyes follow the ball; your body effortlessly and easily reaches up and follows through, as the ball smashes into your opponent's court for an ace. You are focused, sure, and feeling strong.

Now, we will focus on what will happen during your game.

What will you say to yourself during your match to keep you motivated and focused?

Examples could be; stay focused, you got this, you are strong, stay calm.

Pick one that works for you, and say this affirmation to yourself now, silently with conviction.

Take a moment to visualize what you want to happen today and how you want to perform. Imagine every shot you take is executed with perfection. You are playing a flawless match. Every shot you take goes exactly where you want it to. Your forehand, backhand, volleys, and drop shots are perfectly executed. Everyone on your team is in their zone and performing at their very best as well.

You are ready to perform and ready to win. You are ready to show everyone what you are made of and how skilled your team is!

Bring your attention back to an inhalation and an exhalation.

When you are ready, you may open your eyes.

Visualization Two

Breathing: Heart and Belly Breathing

Place one hand on your heart and the other on your belly. Continue to breathe normally and naturally as you focus your attention on the pace of your breathing. You should notice that your breathing slows down when your hands are in this position. As you breathe, send kind wishes to yourself. You can say to yourself:

I am strong.
I am confident.
I am proud of who I am.
I am successful.
I am a winner!

After you repeat these affirmations to yourself, you may allow your hands to fall to your sides or rest in your lap.

We will begin the visualization now.

Recalling a Time:

I want you to remember when and why you wanted to play tennis. Can you remember this time? Can you picture the details? Where were you? Who were you with? What was going on around you? Take a moment to recall this special time that you fell in love with tennis and decided that you wanted to play tennis competitively. Soak in the memory and allow it to fill your mind's eye. Let the memory fill you up with joy, energy, positivity, and happiness.

Allow those positive feelings and feelings of determination, motivation, dedication, and drive to fill you up and spread to every part of your being. Soak up all of those wonderful feelings of the time when you first connected with this sport. Now, try to take those wonderful feelings with you in today's match, and have fun participating in this sport.

Now, imagine being on the court right now. I want you to take three long, slow, deep breaths, in through the nose and out through the mouth. Stay in the moment with each breath you take.

You are ready to play today. You will use your breathing to help relax and calm yourself down if you feel you are getting nervous. You will turn your focus inward to get into your zone.

Now, take a moment to see yourself playing a perfect game of tennis. Imagine being in the lead the entire match. Visualize yourself swinging the racket with perfect form and flow, feeling calm and confident in your ability to win this match. What will you say to yourself before you begin your match that will help motivate you today? You want to think of something quick and easy to say, for instance; I've got this, I know this game well, stay calm and cool, focus, smooth swing. Choose a phrase or word that works for you, and I want you to picture yourself on the court before your match, and saying this to yourself before your game begins.

You are ready to perform and ready to win. You are ready to show everyone what you are made of and how skilled your team is!

Remember to breathe. Stop and take five breaths if you need to at any point during the match.

Visualization Three

Breathing: Elephant Breath

Standing tall, take a big deep breath in, as you raise your arms above you, and as you exhale, you let your arms swing between your legs like an elephant's trunk, letting the head and neck go. Roll up like a rag doll. Do this at least five times.

Visualize Your Game:

Imagine that your body is in tip-top condition today.

You feel great!

You are sending positive energy to all of your muscles and body parts.

Imagine and feel that everything is flowing, and you are ready physically for this match.

Imagine yourself on the court today and starting your warm-up.

Imagine your routine and what you will say to yourself to pump yourself up with positivity.

Imagine your warm-up going very well.

Now, imagine being on the tennis court, and you are aware of the other people around you, and the people in the crowd. You can hear soft voices coming from spectators, but none of this matters to you, because you are focusing your attention on hitting, practicing, and warming up.

Imagine your swing feels smooth and strong.
Feel your perfect form and flow while warming up.
Your footwork and agility are on point and accurate. Your movement on the court is quick.
You are in your zone, not letting distractions break your focus.
It feels natural and easy for you to perform.
Imagine swinging with ease, focus, and strength.
You are now warmed up and ready to perform at the top of your game.
You will let mistakes go easily and move on quickly.
You will let nothing stand in your way of performing well.
You will stay focused.
You will succeed in the sport you love!
Bring your attention back to your breathing, focusing on an inhalation and an exhalation.
When you are ready, you may open your eyes.

Visualization Four

Breathing Exercise:

Let's start out by bringing your attention to your breath. Let's see if you can focus on each inhale and each exhale. Can you notice where you are feeling your breath the most today? Do you feel the air moving in and out of your nostrils, or can you feel your chest rise and fall as you breathe, or maybe you notice your belly rising and falling as you breathe? Pick one of these three areas where you most naturally and easily feel your breath. Know that your breathing is always here for you as your anchor, grounding and stabilizing you when you need it.

Body Scan:

Next, allow your body to relax and soften. Starting at the top of your head, relax each body part as you work your way down your body. Allow the face to soften, the neck to relax, the shoulders to drop, the chest to release, and the arms and hands to relax. Move around to your back and allow this area to completely let go of tension; the hips begin to soften; the legs begin to release and elongate, and the feet and toes begin to let go. Your entire body should be completely relaxed and ready to focus on our visualization for today.

Set the Scene:

I want you to create a picture in your mind of the tennis courts you practice on every day. Picture the details of this court, and imagine you are standing on the court admiring the scenery. You feel confident, important, and proud when you compete. Take a moment to allow those great feelings, and the feelings of excitement to spread throughout your whole body.

Now, imagine you are getting ready to enter the courts with your teammates. You are pumped up, excited, eager, full of energy, and positivity. You are ready to compete and perform well.

Now, you are ready to make your entrance. You walk over to the courts with your teammates, and you are ready to start your warm-up. Visualize your warm-up going smoothly and exactly the way you want it to. Your body feels loose, relaxed, and ready to play great tennis. Take a moment to imagine feeling strong, efficient, precise, and ready to perform at your best.

You know this sport, your body knows this sport, and your heart knows this sport. You love to play tennis, and you love to play it well. Feel yourself getting into your zone where you are unstoppable, unbeatable, and unbreakable. Feel confident in your ability as an athlete, feel strong in your presence, feel grounded in your body and mind.

This is your moment to shine; this is your match to claim; this is your time to achieve success. Feel it, believe it, and allow it!

Bring your focus to your breathing. Notice the air coming into the nostrils and the air leaving the nostrils. Take one big deep breath in and release. When you are ready, you may open your eyes.

GLOSSARY

1. Bird-dog - Strengthens the core. Come to all fours and have your knees under hips and hands under shoulders. Extend your right leg back and your left arm forward, reaching with the fingers and toes. Inhale, and as you exhale, draw your right knee in to touch your left elbow and then extend again. Repeat 3-4 times on each side.

2. Bow pose- Lie on your belly and bend your knees, reach around to grab your ankles with your hands. Flex your feet and press your ankles into your hands as you lift your upper torso off the ground. The chest opens, and shoulders roll back for a mini upper body backbend.

3. Butterfly - Soles of the feet together in a seated position. Try to lean forward, reaching with your hands on the ground for an inner thigh stretch.

4. Camel pose – Sit with your buttocks on your heels. Lift up so that your knees are under your hips, and your shins are resting on the floor. Place your hands on your low back. Begin by slowly leaning back, pressing your hips forward for a backbend. When you are ready, reach back with your right hand and try to grab your right ankle; then, reach back with your left hand and try to grab your left ankle. Tilt your head back for a backbend.

5. Cat cow - In table-top position, inhale, as you drop your belly and lift your chin. Exhale, as you round your back and bring your chin to your chest.

6. Chair pose - Stand with your knees and feet together, squeezing your inner thighs, bend your knees and sit back into an imaginary chair with your weight on your heels. Bring your arms up parallel to your ears.

7. Child's pose – Sit with your buttocks on your heels, reaching your arms and hands out in front of you on the ground. Try to lean your buttocks towards your heels, as you reach forward as far as you can with your hands.

8. Cow pose - On all fours in table-top position. As you inhale, drop your belly and lift your chin, shoulders roll back, and your head is looking up.

9. Crescent lunge – One leg is forward with the knee bent at a 90-degree angle, and the other leg is extended and straight back, resting on the toes with the heel off the ground. Arms are parallel to your ears reaching up, and you will feel a stretch in your hip flexor.

10. Dancers pose – Shift your weight onto your left foot, lift your right leg behind you, and with your right hand, grab the top of the foot or ankle. Stretch your left arm up parallel to your ear, and begin to lean forward, pressing your foot into your hand, as you reach out and lower your left arm until it is parallel with the ground. This is a balance pose. Hold for ten seconds. Repeat on the other side.

11. Dancing cat - In table-top position, begin to move your torso in slow circles in one direction, and then switch directions to

open up and stretch the upper back. Make sure to keep your shoulders and hips still.

12. Double pigeon – In a seated position, stack your legs, with each ankle aligned with each knee. Flex the feet and begin to lean forward slightly, reaching your arms out as far as you can. This pose opens your hips.

13. Downward dog - Hands on the ground shoulder-width apart; step the feet back hip-width apart; the body is in a V; head between your arms; press your hips up and reach the tailbone up; press your chest towards your thighs.

14. Eagles pose – Shift your weight to the left foot, take your right leg and wrap it over the left knee, with toes pointing down. If you can, wrap the right foot behind the left leg while maintaining balance. Take the right arm and cross over the left arm, bend at the elbows, and hands are back to back or palms touching. Bend your left knee at a 90-degree angle. Chest is open, shoulders are away from the ears. Hold for five seconds. Repeat on the other side.

15. Figure four (reclined pigeon)- Lay on your back, place your right ankle on your left knee. Grab below your left knee and pull it into you. Also, aim your right knee away from your body for a hip, buttock, and outer thigh stretch. Repeat on the other side.

16. Frog pose - Start on all fours in table-top position. Widen the distance between the knees as much as you can without straining and bring your forearms to the ground and breathe.

17. Half Camel - Kneel on your shins, with knees under hips and hands at your low back, begin to press hips forward and arch

your back. If you want to go further, reach your left hand down for your left ankle, and then return to starting position. Next, reach your right hand down for your right ankle, and look back, and return to starting position.

18. Half lift – Start in a forward fold, as you inhale, lift your upper torso up, parallel to the floor with a straight back, hands slide along your shins. As you exhale, reach your arms and hands towards the ground for a forward fold.

19. Half-moon balance- Shift weight onto the right foot and lift your left leg up so that it is parallel with the floor. Hands are placed flat on the ground. Straighten your right leg and then take your right hand and move it out three inches to the right side while you lift your left arm up to the ceiling. Your body should be facing the left side while you try to balance in this position. Repeat on the other side.

20. Half-moon - Stand with your knees and feet together, squeeze your inner thighs, bring your arms above your head, parallel to your ears, and interlace your fingers. Pointer fingers are touching together. As you inhale, reach up as far as you can, and as you exhale, lean your body to the right as you squeeze your inner thighs together, and keep your chest and chin lifted.

21. Happy baby – Lay on your back, bend your knees and bring them into your belly. Grip the outsides of your feet with your hands and open your knees slightly. Position each ankle directly over the knee, so that your shins are perpendicular to the floor. Flex your feet, and gently press down on your feet. You may rock side to side as you continue to press your knees into your belly.

22. Hero pose – Sit on the ground with your buttocks between your legs. Your feet are on each side of your buttocks. This is to stretch the quads, so when you are ready, you can begin to lean back as far as you can on your elbows or lay all the way down if you can.

23. High plank - Hands are placed under your shoulders on the ground, feet are hip-width apart, resting on the toes, body is parallel to the floor, core is tight and firm.

24. Lizard pose (low lunge forearm stretch) – Step your right leg forward at a 90-degree angle, place hands to the inside of the right foot, and straighten your back leg as best you can, resting on the toes. If you can, try to lower your forearms down to the ground. Let the right leg fan out to the side. Repeat on the other side.

25. Low runners lunge - Right leg is bent with your knee directly over your ankle at a 90-degree angle; hands are on either side of your right foot; your left leg is extended on the floor, with your knee and the top of your foot resting on the ground. Continue to press your hip down towards the floor.

26. Mountain - Stand tall with your feet hip-width apart; arms parallel to your ears, drop your shoulders away from your ears.

27. Pigeon pose - Sit on your right buttocks with your foot close to your groin. Your left leg extended long behind you with the top of the foot resting on the floor. Make sure hips are square and are facing forward. Place your hands on the ground in front of you and sit up tall. Next, begin to lean forward and reach your arms out in front of you on the floor as far as you can.

28. Pike stretch - Seated position with both legs straight in front of you with toes pointing up. Inhale, as you reach arms up to the ceiling, and exhale, as you lean forward, trying to reach your hands towards your toes.

29. Puppy pose – In a table-top position with your knees stacked under your hips, and hands under your shoulders; begin sitting back with your buttocks leaning towards your heels, as you reach your arms out in front of you as far as you can for a chest and shoulder stretch. Make sure your tummy does not rest on your thighs, or your buttocks rest on your heels.

30. Pyramid pose - Stand with your right leg forward and your left leg back about a few feet apart; both legs should be straight; hips are square and facing forward. Inhale, as you reach arms up parallel to your ears; exhale, as you lean forward over your front leg, reaching for either your shin, calf, or ankle to feel a hamstring stretch in your front leg. Press back to feel an extra stretch.

31. Reverse table - Sit with your knees bent and feet flat on the floor hip-width apart; your hands behind you, shoulder-width apart with your fingers facing your feet. Inhale, and as you exhale, press into your feet, lift your buttocks off the ground, lift your hips, and roll your shoulders back as you look back. The body should be parallel to the floor.

32. Reverse warrior - Assume your warrior two position with your legs 4-5 feet apart; your front leg is bent at a 90-degree angle, and your back leg is as extended and straight as you can get it. Turn your back foot out slightly. Align your front heel with the middle of your back foot. Arms lift so that they are parallel

to the floor, reaching with the fingers. Inhale, and as you exhale, begin sliding your backhand along your back leg while you reach up to the ceiling with your front arm. Eyes follow the rising hand.

33. Runners lunge - Bend front leg at a 90-degree angle, so that knee is over the ankle; bring your hands flat on the floor to either side of the front foot. The back leg is as extended and straight as you can get it with the knee off the floor and resting on the toes.

34. Scorpion pose - Lay on the stomach with the arms out like a T, resting on the floor; bend your right knee and then lift the right leg up first, and then begin to lower the leg and cross the leg over to your left, trying to reach your right foot to the ground. Your hips come off the ground, and you are resting on the outside of your leg, stretching the low back and hip. Repeat on the other side

35. Side angle pose - Stand with your feet four-five feet apart and bend your front right leg into a lunge position at a 90-degree angle. Your back leg is straight. Take your right forearm and place it on your right thigh as you lift your left arm towards the ceiling. Try to look up at your hand. You should feel an opening on your entire left side body. Repeat on the other side.

36. Single bow pose - On all fours, extend right arm out in front and left leg behind, reaching with the fingers and toes. Bend the leg and reach around with the right hand to grab the foot. Flex the foot, and as you exhale, press the foot into your hand for a stretch. Repeat on the other side.

37. Shoulder bridge - Lay on your back with your knees bent and feet flat on the floor hip-width apart; place your arms under your body and interlace your fingers so that your shoulders are touching the ground. Straighten your arms as best you can. When you are ready, press into your feet, lift your hips off the ground and roll your shoulders back. You should be resting on your feet and your shoulders.

38. Shoulder stand - In a seated position, roll like a ball backward as you lift your legs off the ground, and straighten them to the ceiling. Bring your hands to your hips to hold yourself up, and your upper arms are resting on the floor supporting you. Legs are straight with your toes pointed. Hold for ten seconds.

39. Spinal balance - On all fours, extend your right leg back and extend your left arm forward, reaching with the fingers and toes. Hold for five seconds and repeat on the other side.

40. Standing leg split - Place your weight on your right foot and place both hands to the ground on either side of the foot. Lift your left leg as high in the air as you can while you try to draw your hands in towards your foot for an extra stretch. Repeat on the other side.

41. Straddle stretch - Seated position with legs far apart. Sit up tall as you inhale, and then, as you exhale, try to lean forward as far as you can, reaching your hands to the ground.

42. Table-top - On your hands and knees, with your knees under your hips and your hands under your shoulders.

43. Thread the needle – come into a table-top position with the hands under your shoulders and your knees under your hips. Place your right arm under your left, reaching the shoulder and

the ear down to the floor for an upper back and shoulder stretch. Repeat on the other side.

44. Tree pose – Shift your weight on one foot as you bring the opposite foot to either the lower shin or upper leg of the standing leg. Press the foot into the inner leg as you turn the knee out to the side, parallel to the floor; bring your hands to heart position with your palms touching.

45. Triangle pose - Stand with your feet four feet apart, front foot facing forward, and back foot turned in slightly. Raise your arms parallel to the floor, reaching with your fingers. Hinge, or lean forward with your upper body from the waist over your front leg. Windmill the arms so that your front hand reaches for your shin or the floor, and your back arm reaches up towards the ceiling. Eyes follow your rising hand.

46. Twisting chair – Stand with your knees and feet together, squeezing your inner thighs; bend your knees, and sit back into an imaginary chair. Bring your hands to the heart center, with the palms touching. Twist your upper torso to your right, and place your left elbow on the outside of your right knee. Continue to twist to the right. Repeat on the other side.

47. Upward dog - Lay on your stomach; place hands by your sides at chest level with palms flat on the floor; press into your palms, and slowly lift your upper torso and hips off the ground; chin lifts, as you drop the shoulders, and rest the tops of the feet on the floor.

48. Warrior One – Step the right leg forward and bend it at a 90-degree angle; the left leg is extended and straight behind you. Make sure your left foot is turned out slightly, square your hips

forward, and reach arms up parallel to your ears. This is a hip-opening stretch for the back leg. Repeat on the other side.

49. Warrior Two - Step your feet about four feet apart and bring your arms parallel to the floor, reaching out with your fingers. Turn your back foot out slightly, and make sure to align your front heel with the middle of your back foot. Bend your front leg at a 90-degree angle, and your back leg is extended and firm. Eyes look over your front middle finger.

50. Warrior Three – Shift your weight onto your right foot, bring your left leg up, parallel to the floor, big toe facing the floor, and press your heel away. Hands at your sides as you look forward and balance. Repeat on the other side.

51. Wide leg forward bend - Stand with feet four-five feet apart, with your hands on your hips, and a straight back. Lower yourself down and place your hands flat on the floor with your legs wide. Try to place your weight on the balls of your feet for an extra hamstring stretch in both legs.

52. Wide child's pose – Sit with your buttocks on your heels. Your knees are about one-two feet apart; extend your arms and hands forward, as you sit back into your heels.

53. Windshield wipers - Lay on your stomach, with your head resting on your hands, bend your knees, and let your lower legs rock side to side to loosen the low back.

REFERENCES

Biegel, G. M., & Corbin, T. H. (2018). Mindfulness for Student Athletes. New Harbinger Publications.

Burdick, D. (2014). Mindfulness Skills for Kids & Teens. A Workbook for Clinicians & Clients with 154 Tools, Techniques, Activities & Worksheets. PESI Publishing & Media.

Fletcher, J. (2019, February 12). How to use 4-7-8 Breathing for Anxiety. Medical News Today. https://www.medicalnewstoday.com/articles/324417

Guber, T., Kalish, L., Fatus, S. (2005). Yoga Pretzels: 50 Fun Activities for Kids & Grownups Cards. Barefoot Books. Yoga Ed.

Harper, J.C., Gonzalez, M., Gonzalez, A., & Gilmour, K. (2017). Yoga & Mindfulness Practices for Teens Card Deck. PESI Publishing & Media. Little Flower Yoga.

Mayo Clinic Health System (2020, June 6). 5,4,3,2,1: Countdown to Make Anxiety Blast Off. https://www.mayoclinichealthsystem.org/hometown-health/speaking-of-health/5-43-2-1countdown-to-make-anxiety-blast-off

Meggyesy, D. (2016, February 22). 90% Mental, 10% Physical:The Inner Game. The Sports, Energy, and Consciousness Group. http://sportsenergygroup.com/90-mental-10-physical-the-inner-game-by-david-meggyesy/

Mindfulness Exercises. (2021). Free Guided Meditation Scripts. https://mindfulnessexercises.com/free-guided-meditation-scripts/

Mindful Schools. (2015). https://www.mindfulschools.org/

Saltzman, A. (2018). A Still Quiet Place for Athletes. New Harbinger Publications.

Stone, A. M. (2019, November 19). 90 Seconds to Emotional Resilience. https://www.alysonmstone.com/90-seconds-to-emotional-resilience/#:~:text=%E2%80%9CWhen%20a%20person%20has%20a,stay%20in%20that%20emotional%20loop.%E2%80%9D

Yoga Stick figure Images. (© 2021). Yoga By Design. yogabydesign.com.au

www.ingramcontent.com/pod-product-compliance
Lightning Source LLC
Chambersburg PA
CBHW061559110426
42742CB00038B/1588